Praise for
C H O O S e Peace *&* Happiness

"Simple directives bring profound results. Follow the
guidelines in this wonderful book!"

—EVe ELIOT, author of *Attention Shoppers!*

"Susyn Reeve gives us a map to peace and happiness—to
truly BE peace and happiness. With her guidance this
is possible, no matter what your situation may be. Allow
this marvelous book to show you the way."

—SanDY VILaS, CEO of CoachInc.com
and author of *Power Networking*

"There is so much offered in Susyn Reeve's
Choose Peace & Happiness that it could even
be the basis for a musical!"

—RICHarD ADLer, lyricist and composer; Broadway
shows include *The Pajama Game* and *Damn Yankees*

"Gain important insights by practicing the simple yet
empowering "peace and happiness" exercises in this
nurturing and motivational book. The restorative
awakenings you will experience are invaluable."

—MonTe FarBer and AMY zerner, authors of
*Love, Light, and Laughter; Gifts of the Goddess
Affirmation Cards;* and *The Healing Deck*

D1550585

CHOOSE
Peace &
Happiness

A 52-Week Guide

To: Janine
Be Peace & Happiness
Smile - Hug -
Be the world's Greatest
Lover!
With love,
Susyn

SUSYN REEVE

Red Wheel
Boston, MA / York Beach, ME

In memory of my Mom
Ethel Schlesinger
Your love keeps lifting me higher

First published in 2003 by
Red Wheel/Weiser, LLC
York Beach, ME
With offices at:
368 Congress Street
Boston, MA 02210
www.redwheelweiser.com

A percentage of the author's proceeds from the sale of this book will be donated to the Sixth Sun
Foundation, a non-profit organization dedicated to empowering people to transform their lives
through the teachings brought forth by don Miguel Ruiz (www.sixthsunfoundation.org), and the
M.K. Gandhi Institute for Nonviolence promoting and applying the principles of nonviolence
locally, nationally, and globally (www.gandhiinstitute.org).

Library of Congress Cataloging-in-Publication Data

Reeve, Susyn.
    Choose peace & happiness : a 52-week guide / Susyn Reeve.
        p. cm.
    ISBN 1-59003-059-1
    1. Peace of mind—Problems, exercises, etc. 2. Happiness—Problems,
exercises, etc. I. Title: Choose peace and happiness. II. Title.
    BF637.P3R44 2003
    646.7—dc21   2003008573

Typeset in Filosofia and Bliss by Suzanne Albertson.

TCP

10 09 08 07 06 05 04
 8 7 6 5 4 3 2

contents

CHOOSE Peace & Happiness

preface

Be the change you wish to see in the world.
—MAHATMA,GANDHI

I began writing this book in August 2001, after I had been asked to design a workshop focusing on peace and happiness for employees at Mount Sinai NYU Health (a large medical center in New York City with more than twenty thousand employees). It seemed to me that, in addition to a workshop, this topic would lend itself to a simple guidebook that could be used to develop new patterns of thought and behavior to reinforce the experience of peace and happiness in everyday life.

Then the startling events of September 11 occurred. The room in my house with the TV was being painted and the TV was unplugged, so I spent most of September 12 and 13 gardening. I learned much from seeing how some plants exist effortlessly side by side with their roots entangled while other plants strangle each other when they are too close together. I saw my garden transform when I gave plants more breathing space. In the midst of this, at times, I felt helpless. I was 120 miles from New York City, not knowing what to do to help other than sending money. At other times I thought that being in my garden, listening to many versions of *Amazing Grace* on my CD player, was my greatest contribution to peace on earth. Feeling peace within me during a time of fear and terror in the world was the most powerful gift I could give to myself and to the collective consciousness of the planet. I wrote the following letter to the *East Hampton Star*, one of my local newspapers:

WHAT IF?

What if there was peace on earth—what would it look like? How would we know it? Peace is not simply the absence of war—it is a way of being. And if we don't begin practicing that way of being, how can there ever really be peace? As the song says: "Let there be peace on earth and let it begin with me."

I am an Interfaith minister. I have studied the spiritual foundations of the world religions. What I have come to know through my studies, my fifty-two years of life experience, and my thirty years of teaching human relations skills to individuals and in organizations is that in their heart of hearts, all people want peace. Some see war as the way to peace, some see meditation as the way to peace, some see meditation and prayer as the way to peace, some see nonviolence as the way to peace, some see the Golden Rule as the way to peace. While we may see different means we all speak of the same end: A peaceful and loving world.

Well, how do we get it? My point of view is simple. It is reflected in this quote by Gandhi, "Be the change you wish to see in the world." Another way of saying this is from the New Thought religion: "Thoughts held in mind manifest over time." I believe that the thoughts we think, fueled by our passion and desire, acted on with conviction, and voiced with authority, create the world that we live in. *In the beginning was the word, and the word was with God, and the word was God.* God is the creative force in the universe, and our word is our creative force in our world. What if we begin, as individuals, families, coworkers, a nation, a world community, to focus our thoughts on peace? What if, for one minute each night at 9:00 P.M. EST, we focus our loving attention on peace? What if during the week of Thanksgiving all TV programs, all radio, all national and international media focus on peace? What if, starting today, we each live our lives as an example of peace, as if our life depends on it, for truly it does?

How do we do this? Be conscious of your language, practice for-giveness, express gratitude, express your love, lend a helping hand, talk about peace with your family, friends, and coworkers, smile, hug, ask for help, give help, respect differences, live each moment as if it is a precious gift, practice "The Four Agreements" from the book by the same name by don Miguel Ruiz.

- Be impeccable with your word.
- Don't take things personally.
- Don't make assumptions.
- Always do your best.

What if through the wake-up call of September 11, 2001, the words of John Lennon came to life: "Imagine all the people living life in peace. You may say I'm a dreamer, but I'm not the only one. I hope someday you'll join us and the world will be as one."

It is now March 24, 2003, and war is being waged in Iraq. In the midst of this war the voice for peace is being heard throughout the world. And while current reality looks as though peace is a distant ideal, I know that the more each individual in the world lives a daily life of kindness, compassion, and love—in their homes, on line at the supermarket, in the workplace, in traffic, in the midst of personal challenges, during each moment of the day—we are changing the world. When I notice I am angry and abusive to myself or others, I stop, take a deep breath, and remember that we truly are all connected in this mysterious adventure known as life. I can choose in the moment to be peace and happiness and breathe that reality into three-dimensional life on earth.

So this book is more than a simple guide. While the ideas and techniques described in it are simple to do, the impact of each one of us creating a personal experience of peace truly can create peace on earth. Peace begins with an idea, fueled by our desire, acted on with conviction, and spoken of with authority. This book is an invitation to you to add your energy to the collective consciousness of peace on earth.

Inner Peace

Notes on Inner Peace and Spiritual Growth
ELSA JOY BAILEY

There is no surprise like the surprise of Inner Peace: it's as startling as a moonbeam visible at high noon. How it operates is beyond me: I only know it is reliable if I am reliable—if I remember to stop and call to it when the trees are upside down and the birds have quit singing.

Inner Peace is reliable and it is spiritual food, yet there's nothing routine about it, ever. Time after time I have paused to call on Inner Peace when I had no idea what shape it would take and what it might say when it got there. Inner Peace has, in fact, no standard answers—have you noticed that? It is as unpredictable as jumping beans. All we can observe is that when we do open the door to invite it in—it is always right on the money, always perfect in its response.

I remember a particular day when everything in life seemed to be going awry. Somehow I had tumbled deep into a pool of disorder. To say it another way, I found myself looking at things as they seemed and no further. How they seemed was chaotic. So it went along in this manner for a while, me walking on slippery ground, until out of nowhere I suddenly felt an impulse toward sanity.

The impulse settled on me like a friendly hand, straightening my wind-blown cap with a quick tap. Following that tap, I spent an entire day meditating on order, on peace. I made it my day's work. Putting everything human, everything me aside, I simply called to Inner Peace. And called to it. And called to it. And what happened during that day? Nothing. But, by the next morning, all the world seemed slower and softer and less dangerous. Mysteriously, I began cleaning out closets and neatening the house. Something heavy had lifted out of my awareness. And in its place, there it was: a subtle but tangible No-Thing with its own faint fragrance and a distinct hum: Inner Peace.

No, I don't know how it does that, but it does. It floats into our presence like a surprise summer mist. Moistening the dry spots. Calming the tides. Combing the tangles. Feeding the hungers. I've seen it come a thousand and one times, and still it is a mystery. It probably always will be. All I know is, without it, I'm nothing.

acknowledgments

With heartfelt thanks and appreciation may you feel the love I am sending your way. Robin Cohen, thank you for the phone call asking me to lead a workshop for Mount Sinai Medical Center employees on peace and happiness. You provided the topic that my heart and mind responded to with a resounding YES. Eve Eliot, my first friend in East Hampton, thank you for helping me "grok" that I could do it. Amy Zerner and Monte Farber for your friendship, belief in me, and the introduction to Jan Johnson. My weekly Being Peace & Happiness email list, your saying yes to receiving weekly emails kept me on track with a new chapter to send out each week. Susan Ivory, thank you for reading each word, eliminating all those unnecessary "thats," and being an example of the power of choosing peace and happiness. To The Ladies Pajama Party Group who journeyed with me when I questioned if peace and happiness were possible for me and who celebrate with me now that I am peace and happiness. To Byll and Dan who have loved me and opened the door for me to love me. To Mary Angela Buffo and Lindsey Kane: thank you for inviting me to co-create Love's Way Spiritual Circle and give voice to the loving energy of the universe expressed through me. Robin and Mark Neiman, thanks for the invitation to Silva Mind Control in 1972 and your love ever since. Joan and Bruce Breiner, you are my anchors and reminders to celebrate somebody. Shanti, thanks for sharing the journey.

To my teachers and mentors along the way, your influence, encouragement, wisdom, and humor is alive in the pages of this book. To don Miguel Ruiz, thank you for the invitation to heaven on earth and the faith to jump fully into life on earth. To the Dreamers, I am blessed by your radiant presence. And to Lorraine Simone, sister of my spirit, Ah Ho.

A special thanks to the thousands of students, workshop participants, and friends who have given me the opportunity to share and expand my work by allowing me into their lives. And to the members of Mount Sinai NYU Health who have given me limitless opportunities to fine-tune my instrument: you are the best.

To my Red Wheel Weiser partners in birthing this book: Jan Johnson, your enthusiasm about my book proposal woke up every cell in my being; Jill Rogers, your voice on the phone is a comfort; and Robyn Heisey, your purple emails are energizing and tap my creative juices; and the Project Design team, you've captured the essence beautifully.

To the children in my life Maya, Adam, David, Gabriel, Gabriele, Lyssa, Nina, Lara, Solange, Troy, both Kevins, Tim, and Dwayne, this is for you, your children, and all the children.

And always, the still small voice within, thank you for speaking loud enough for me to hear and clear enough for me to understand.

INTRODUCTION

What do we want? Happiness. When do we want it? Now, if not yesterday. And yet how many people do you know who actually experience happiness and peace regularly as a way of being? Who pops into your mind? Are you on this list? If you are reading this right now, you are probably hoping this book will finally have your key to open the door to peace and happiness in your life.

So let's begin. Are you sure you're ready for it? Do you really want it? Are you ready to experience peace and happiness in your life? If you want to experience peace and happiness, you have to be peace and happiness, starting in your thoughts and manifested through your actions. You may be thinking, "Well, if I knew how to do that, I wouldn't be reading this book."

Here's how you do it. It begins with a choice. Peace and happiness begin as a point of view through which you see and experience the world. So if you want it, choose it. Know that right now all the power that ever was and ever will be is available to you. You can tap into this power and choose peace and happiness, knowing that by making this choice you open a door to the experience of heaven on earth.

This is powerful. So, a cautionary note: once you make this choice, it is possible that in glimpsing what you have asked for, you may also experience some distress, turmoil, pain, sadness, and depression. This is natural and normal. It simply means all of your personal blocks and obstacles to being peace and happiness are coming to the surface of your conscious awareness. When your resistance comes to the light of your awareness, you can acknowledge it and let it go. It is as if by making the choice for peace and happiness, you are making the choice to clean house, and you have not cleaned house for many years, or you have not done a thorough job. You simply moved things from one place to another. Know if you have already lived with the discomfort of stress and fear in your life, you will be able to move through the discomfort of this change, and in the process, you will be consciously creating new patterns of thought that will result in the happiness, peace, and love in your daily life that you yearn for. If you ever feel scared or alone, ask for help.

- Talk with a friend
- Talk to God

- Talk with a counselor or coach
- Contact me at *www.SusynReeve.com*

So are you ready for the most glorious adventure of your life? I know you can do it because I've done it. Read and follow the instructions below:

1. Make yourself comfortable, preferably sitting, with your feet flat on the floor, your spine straight, your arms resting gently on your thighs, with this book opened to the "Prayer for Peace and Happiness" on page 3.
2. Close your eyes.
3. Breathe. Inhale through your nose, deeply and fully, a sense of peace and happiness. As you exhale, through your mouth, relax into the loving embrace of the universe, feeling yourself fully and gently supported by the chair you are sitting on. Repeat this five times.
4. Open your eyes, read aloud the "Prayer for Peace and Happiness" on page 3, allowing this message to fill your being as you focus your attention on each word.

Prayer For
Peace and Happiness

Today, with heartfelt gratitude, I live my life through the experience of peace and happiness. I easily focus my attention on thoughts that enhance the flow of love in my life. I know I create my experience through the point of view I choose. Through inviting and allowing peace and happiness, I acknowledge that I am peace, I am happiness, I am love. I ask for and receive all the help available to me, visible and invisible, to easily release habit patterns of fear, to have faith in a loving future, and to live as love in the present.

To the eternal peace and happiness of all

—and so it is.

Say this prayer both morning and night, so you breathe life into this idea each day.

HOW TO USE THIS BOOK

This book was written to be used during the course of a year, to expand peace and happiness in your daily life. I suggest that you take your time with it. While you may want to read it from cover to cover, to receive its greatest value, combine the ideas with action. And as we all know walking the talk requires action, and practice is the method to create peace and happiness habits and patterns in your daily thoughts and behavior.

Here are three ways to use this book. You can choose one or use the combination that works best for you.

One: Start at the beginning and focus on one chapter per week. There are 52 ideas, one for each week. Each idea then has 7 days of techniques and exercises for you to practice, one for each day of the week. Day 7 includes writing your reflections, which you can do in your own journal if you have one already or in a separate journal you use just with this book (see Week 3 on journaling).

I am aware that some people love having a clear structure and will easily follow the exercises in the order they are given, while others will prefer to have more choice in deciding the order of exercises, or even which of the seven days of how-tos to do. What is most important is to practice and experiment with the exercises described. Being peace and happiness involves both having a conceptual understanding of the ideas involved *and* putting them into action in your life.

Two: Each day open the book at random and implement an exercise related to the idea in that chapter. Before you actually open the book identify your intention.

- I choose to have my highest guidance for today in being peace and happiness.
- Guide me in how best to deal with (identify whatever circumstance or situation is on your mind).
- Show me the way.

Three: Use the book in a group. Plan to meet for an hour or two. Invite friends to meet weekly, in person, on the phone, in an email chat; or if you lead personal development groups as part of your work, form a group using *Choose Peace and Happiness* as the material you base your weekly sessions on. Plan to meet for an hour or two. Either way, as an informal peace and happiness support group or a professional group, you may structure each session in the following format.

Start the session by saying aloud the "Prayer for Peace and Happiness" (see page 3).

Identify ground rules. Some examples are: Start and end on time. Let someone know if you do not plan to attend. Do the reading and practice the exercises. One person talks at a time. Keep the focus on your patterns of thoughts and behavior and how they contribute to or detract from being peace and happiness; not on how other people *should* be different or are the cause of your problems. Support others in identifying their patterns of thought and behavior rather than giving advice. Ask for help when you need it. Have fun.

Use the Be Here Now technique for relaxation. Have each person write down all the things that are cluttering his or her mind right now. Include chores to complete and questions you have. As you write each item down, know that you are clearing your mind to be more fully present here and now. When everyone has completed their list, put it aside knowing that you may add to it as the group goes on and that your mind is clear to receive the greatest benefit from the group.

To further relax and open to a deeper listening and receptivity, one member of the group can lead you through the following guided visualization: Sit comfortably. Close your eyes. As I count from one to five, focus on your breath as you inhale a sense of calm and relaxation through your nose and exhale completely through you mouth. At the count of five, experience yourself as more relaxed and at ease, ready to expand your experience of peace and happiness. **One**, continuing to focus on your breath. Breathing in a sense of calm and relaxation and exhaling completely. **Two**, if you notice any tension or tightness in your body, breathe into that part of your body and as you exhale experience yourself as more relaxed, more at ease. **Three**, if thoughts enter your mind, simply notice them, and as you exhale let them go, continuing to focus your attention on your breath, breathing in a deeper sense of calm and relaxation and exhaling completely. **Four**, continuing to focus on your breath as you allow yourself to fully relax your mind and body, feeling a sense of renewal filling your being. And **Five**, experiencing yourself as relaxed and alert. Fully supported by the seat beneath you. Allowing peace and happiness to fill your being as you now open yourself to deepening your experience of peace and happiness. And taking a deep breath, identify a powerful peace and happiness experience you had during the past week. And now as you feel yourself fully present here and now, allow your eyes to open, feeling wide awake, alert, better than before.

Then have each person report a powerful peace and happiness experience he or she had this week. (At your first group meeting, have people share why they are joining the group at this time.) You may choose to go around the circle a few times and address the following items:

- Describe your most powerful peace and happiness experience this week.
- What was your experience with the exercises?
- How are you going to continue to use last week's idea in your daily life?

Agree on a specific time frame for this reporting, for instance, fifteen minutes for all group members to share. Otherwise, you may notice that suddenly an hour has gone by. While it is important to use a structure, if there is some topic that generates a strong reaction you may decide to focus on it, and if you do, check with the members of the group to see if focusing on the issue that has come up would be helpful to them now. *Caution:* stories take a long time to tell and your focus is to identify patterns of thought rather than hearing the on-going saga!

Read aloud the chapter for the coming week. One person can read it, or each person can read a paragraph—experiment. I recommend that each person read the week's material before the group meets and that one person in the group be the "leader" for the discussion. The "leader" will prepare questions that relate to the chapter and may also come in with a list of resources. Sample "leader" questions:

- What is your understanding of this idea?
- How does this idea relate to being peace and happiness?
- Do you currently make use of this idea? If yes, how?
- What challenges do you anticipate in making use of this idea? What support do you need to practice it anyway?

Close by identifying next week's chapter and "leader." End with the group reciting the "Prayer for Peace and Happiness" aloud.

week 1:
Use the Law of Attraction

There seems to be a great law of Nature whereby an atom
attracts to itself that which is needed for its development.
And the force that brings about these results manifests itself in
Desire. There may be many Desires, but the predominant one
has the strongest attracting power. This law is recognized
through the various kingdoms of Nature, but it is only begin-
ning to be realized that the same Law maintains in the king-
dom of the mind.

—WILLIAM WALKER ATKINSON,
THE LAW OF THE NEW THOUGHT

The law of attraction is a universal law and the paradigm for peace and happiness. The idea is quite simple: what you think is what you get. Thoughts fueled with desire (emotional energy), spoken with authority (you are the author!), and acted on with conviction (faith, believing in something one hundred percent) is what you create in your life. This law operates whether or not we are conscious of our thoughts. It is as if the universe hears us through our dominant thoughts and through our vibrations and always responds with a resounding YES. What this means is that all of our life experience begins with us. Everything, every relationship, every event, is first created in our consciousness before it takes form in three-dimensional reality. Each one of us is continually creating our world. Consciously using this knowledge is our point of power. To shift our paradigm requires commitment and discipline, the same kind of discipline and focus of attention you would use if you were training for a marathon. Left to our own devices, most of us get lazy. We tend to follow the path of least resistance, whether or not that path is satisfying.

If you desire a deeper and more consistent experience of peace and happiness in your life, then your dominant thoughts must reflect your desire. When we have a strong desire for something, we are used to *looking* to see if it is there yet. Imbedded in that *looking* is the belief that it isn't there (since if it were there, we wouldn't be looking!). We are so used to giving more power to visible outside circumstances than to the power of our in-visible intention wedded with faith that we often simply don't allow the gifts of the universe into our lives.

Another stumbling block to peace and happiness is that many of us are walking around with beliefs about ourselves that go something like this:

- I'm not good enough.
- I'm not kind enough.
- I'm not smart enough.
- I'm not loveable enough.
- I'm not wealthy enough.
- I'm not strong enough.
- I'm not young enough.
- I'm not thin enough.

We have gathered so much evidence through the years to support our belief that we have faith in it, and the law of attraction goes into high gear, saying YES to our dominant thought. Thereby we create experiences to further support getting what we really don't want.

Rather than deciding if you believe or don't believe in the law of attraction, I invite you to act as if it is true, imagine it is true, and play with it. And if some evidence would help you, think of all those things you have called coincidence or synchronicity—for example, when you think of someone and they seem to call you out of the blue or when you hear about a new book or movie that you'd never heard of before and suddenly the next five people you talk with mention it as well. Or you say you are certain you are not going to get a parking space in the center of town and you don't; or you meet someone and you know within moments that this is the person you'll marry, and now you are married to that person! The truth is the law of attraction has been at work in your life already! What if you truly are made in the image of the creator and you are the artist, the creator of the greatest masterpiece of all: your life? Would you choose heaven rather than hell, peace rather than war, love rather than fear? Make these choices this week and every day and notice peace and happiness taking center stage in your life.

HOW TO DO IT

RESOURCES

~ *The Law of New Thought* by William Walker Atkinson, Pomeroy, WA: Health Research, 1967 (*www.healthresearchbooks.com*).

~ *Stepping into the Aquarian Age* by Nancy Privett,
Westhampton, NY: Old Lion Publishing, 2001.
~ Abraham-Hicks Book and Tapes
(830 755-2299; *www.abraham-hicks.com*).
~ *The Matrix* and the *Matrix Reloaded* (movies).

DAY 1: Play with the law of attraction. Focus on things and people and watch them show up. Imagine loose change in the morning and then spend thirty seconds pretending it is the end of the day and you are telling your family and friends about the loose change you found today. Then let it go, release this idea into the universe like a helium balloon. During the day, loose change will have your name on it. No telling where it will show up: on the street, in your car ashtray that you hadn't opened since you got the car; in your raincoat pocket, inside your wallet. Whenever it shows up, acknowledge it, saying, *"yes, the law of attraction works"* and then the universe will say YES to this idea as well. Play. This format may be helpful:

· Identify something you want to attract.
· Imagine you've attracted it. Create a virtual reality and for thirty
  seconds, visualize your desire realized. Make sure to include yourself
  in the picture and how you feel achieving your results (getting out of
  your car after easily getting a parking space and saying to yourself, "It
  was really easy getting this space," and feeling great about it with a
  smile on your face; sitting in a seat on a crowded subway or bus
  immediately after you've got on it and thinking to yourself, "I'm so
  glad I got this seat" and feeling relaxed and at ease).
· Let it go. Allow the universe to provide with a resounding YES.
· Receive it when it knocks at your door.

DAY 2: Identify what is in your life that is not a source of peace and happiness and focus your attention on what you do want. For example, if your job is unsatisfying and you have spent much of the past six months complaining about it, stop the complaining and imagine you are in a satisfying job. If creating a virtual reality with your boss in it results in anxious feelings, imagine that you are getting home from work and telling your family or friends what a great day you had at work. Let the universe provide the details. You may unexpectedly get a call from a headhunter with a great job interview for you; your boss may be transferred and your new boss is great; or maybe you are offered that position! Have faith that the universe has heard you and let it go. And if all thoughts about work result in feelings of unrest, trust that the universe has heard your desire for a satisfying job and focus your attention on anything that gives you pleasure, because that is the vibration that allows you to be open to the resounding YES of the universe answering your desire.

DAY 3: Any time during the day that you are out of sync with peace and happiness, choose in the moment to attract a new experience.

- *Acknowledge you are feeling yucky.* You have been seduced by abusive and judgmental thoughts about yourself or others. You are feeling victimized and isolated; revenge may be on your mind or guilt has found a comfortable home!
- *Say "oops."* Use your personal power to stop the train of negative thoughts.
- *Choose your desire.* Say aloud (allowed!) or think to yourself: "I choose feeling: (happy, light-hearted, grateful, and so forth) for this moment."
- Let it go and move on. With your attention focused in the present moment, smell the flowers.

DAY 4: Make a pleasure list of things on which you can focus your attention. Carry the list with you, put it on your Palm Pilot, paste it to your refrigerator, and put it by the side of your bed. Use this list to shift your attention when you are attracting hellish experiences into your life. Here are some of my pleasure list items:

- My granddaughter's giggle and the sound of her voice.
- The morning sun, glistening on the ocean, as I walk along the water's edge. My dog playfully romping ahead of me.
- Snuggles with my lover on my couch in front of a roaring fire in the fireplace; getting a foot massage from my lover.
- The full moon lighting the sky.
- The smell of fresh baked bread as I walk into my house on a rainy winter day.
- Hearing my golf club connect with the ball. Seeing the ball soar and land on the green, on a fall afternoon.

DAY 5: Use the law of attraction for the well-being of others. Here are some ways to do it:

- If you have a family member or friend who has been suffering, place his or her photo on your refrigerator and every time you look at the photo, see him as whole and happy; say a prayer for her highest good.
- If you pass a car accident on the road, instead of getting caught up in the horror, say a prayer for the well-being of all involved and express your gratitude for the emergency service workers at the scene. I have noticed that when I do this, rather than getting seduced by the drama, I feel as if I am contributing to the well-being of the people involved as well as to my own. Since I have faith in the power of thought, I know I am contributing to a greater experience of peace and happiness on whatever I am focusing my attention.

DAY 6: Expand the law of attraction to the world. See peace on earth. Imagine a news telecast declaring peace in the Middle East, peace between the United States and Iraq. Use the power of your thought to influence the collective consciousness of the planet. We attract what we put our attention on. This is true in our individual lives, in our families, communities, workplace, countries, and in our world.

DAY 7: Write your reflections on the law of attraction.

- What did you learn about yourself?
- How can you apply this in your daily life? Do it.

Loose Change

When I wrote this chapter, the idea to practice the law of attraction with loose change simply popped into my mind as I wrote the Day 1 exercise. The next morning I went to the gym. When I got on the elliptical trainer to work out there was loose change in the cup holder. The law of attraction popped into my mind. I smiled. After thirty minutes I got off the elliptical trainer and went to a bench to lift free weights. After a few minutes, I realized that I'd left my new-found loose change where I had found it. When I finished using the weights, I was bending down to pick up my towel and I saw more loose change. "Ah yes," I thought, "when I express a desire and let it go, the universe says: YES."

—SR

Ask, and it will be given to you;
Seek, and you will find;
Knock, and it will be opened to you.

—MATTHEW 7:7

WEEK 2:
Acknowledge Accomplishments

When you get to the top of the mountain, your first
inclination is not to jump for joy, but to look around.
—JAMES CARVILLE

Acknowledging accomplishments is an important element of the creative process. In 1982, when I studied with Robert Fritz, author of *The Path of Least Resistance*, I learned about the importance of acknowledging our accomplishments. He described the creative process as having the following three components:

- *Germination*—an inner process where the seed of an idea is planted in the fertile soil of our consciousness (the idea for this book, for example).
- *Assimilation*—when we begin to see the fruits of the seeds we have germinated in our life (a book proposal is written; the proposal is sent to publishers; a book contract is signed; the manuscript is completed and sent to the publisher).
- *Completion*—acknowledgment of the completion of the creation (Yippee! I completed my book proposal; I'm so glad my friends spoke with their publisher about taking a look at my proposal; YES, I have a book contract, thank you, God, Loving Power of the Universe for guiding my way, Hooray! I've completed my manuscript; I am thrilled my book is a bestseller).

He told us that in his research of composers, all had the artistic and technical skills to compose music. The difference between the ones who were successful and the ones who were not was that successful composers went through all three steps of the creative process. Some people had great ideas and stopped there; others had ideas and took action; but it was the people who had ideas, took action, and acknowledged their accomplishments who experienced success.

We feel good when we acknowledge our accomplishments, but many of us are not skilled at doing this. We have more practice focusing our attention

13

on what didn't work or what is left to be done. We acknowledge, but what we acknowledge is what is lacking. Think about it. Have you ever completed ten items on your daily to-do list and found yourself only thinking about the two you didn't complete at the end of the day? This drains our energy. When we focus on and acknowledge our accomplishments, the force is with us. This force gives us the energy to move with grace and ease and at the end of the day, we feel alive and good about who we are. Not only does acknowledging our accomplishments enhance our personal well-being, it contributes loving energy to the collective consciousness of peace and happiness in the world. Each and every moment we have one hundred percent power to choose what we think and where we focus our attention, so acknowledge your accomplishments this week. This is a week for celebration!

HOW TO DO IT

DAY 1: At the end of the day, write down five things you accomplished. Do this every day this week. Do this when you are questioning your ability to get things done or feeling blue. This exercise is less about the content of your items and more about seeing yourself through the eyes of accomplishment. For some of you this will be like wearing new glasses. You may not be used to them at first, but suddenly your vision will clear.

DAY 2: Choose an Accomplishment Symbol (based on Robert Fritz's Symbolic Gesture). An Accomplishment Symbol is something you normally do each day that you endow with the power to represent an accomplishment. Your Accomplishment Symbol may be brushing your teeth, washing your face, shaving, having breakfast, getting out of bed. Remember, it is something you are already doing, NOT something you think you *should* be doing.

Since 1982 my Accomplishment Symbol has been brushing my teeth. The association between accomplishment and brushing my teeth is now so strong that I go to bed and wake up feeling a sense of accomplishment just by brushing my teeth. Even if it is just a glimmer on some days, the energy of accomplishment is still there. There have been some days just getting the toothbrush to my mouth felt like a major effort. I would just wet it a bit, not even use toothpaste, and still I would go to bed thinking, "Well I brushed my teeth today. I accomplished something!"

DAY 3: Use self-talk to acknowledge your accomplishments. You might look in the mirror and say, "Good for me! Today I wrote, exercised at the gym, and prepared the material for the class I am teaching tomorrow." While waiting in line at the supermarket you might say to yourself, "I got a lot done today: I sent a birthday gift to my Mom, I paid my bills, I went to the gym, and I am getting the weekly supermarket shopping done right now." While you are on hold on the phone you might say to yourself, "I've accomplished a lot today: I went to the barber, I saw my son's school play, and I spoke with the mortgage broker about refinancing our mortgage at a lower rate."

DAY 4: Brag to three people about your accomplishments.

DAY 5: Get yourself a treat to celebrate your accomplishments. It may be a bouquet of flowers, that new CD you've wanted, a massage, a tie that makes you smile.

DAY 6: Acknowledge something of value in each encounter you have today. See everything you do today through the eyes of accomplishment. Sometimes, when I am stuck in traffic and on the verge of giving the steering wheel of my life over to impatience, I remind myself of this great opportunity to practice patience, and I acknowledge myself for turning lemons into lemonade. Becoming the greatest lemonade maker in the world is a terrific accomplishment and a sure way to be peace and happiness.

DAY 7: Write your reflections on acknowledging your accomplishments.

- What did you accomplish?
- What did you learn?
- How can you keep your muscle of acknowledging accomplishments firm, strong, and well-toned? Do it.

The Wonderful Cracked Pot

Once there was a man who carried water every day from a stream to his house. He carried it in two large pots hung on each end of a pole slung across his neck. He called them his "wonderful pots."

One pot was perfect. It was always full of water at the end of the long walk from the stream. The other pot was cracked. It leaked, and always arrived at the house only half full. One day by the stream it spoke to the man.

"I am ashamed of myself," it said.

"Why?" the man asked.

"Water leaks out of the crack in my side, all the way back to your house," the pot said. "Because I'm not perfect, you can't bring home two full pots of water. I'm a failure; just a cracked pot."

"You should not feel that way," the man said. "You are not a failure. You are a wonderful pot. And, you can prove it to yourself. As we return to the house today, look carefully alongside the path. When we get home, tell me what you saw."

All the way home, the cracked pot paid attention to everything he saw. At home the man asked, "What did you see?"

"Flowers," said the cracked pot. "I saw lots of flowers."

"Yes you did. Aren't they beautiful?"

"Yes," said the pot. "But, once again, half the water I was carrying leaked out. I'm sorry."

"There is no need to be sorry," said the man. "Tell me, did you notice where the flowers were growing?"

"Well yes," said the pot, a little puzzled. "They were only on my side of the path, but not on the other side. Why is that?"

"For all these years," the man said, "I have planted flower seeds on your side of the path. Every day as we walked back from the stream—"

"Ohhhhh!" the pot interrupted, shaking with excitement. "I watered the seeds through the crack in my side, and the seeds sprouted and the flowers bloomed, and—"

"Yesssss," said the man, who was as excited as the pot. "Because you are the way you are, everyone in the village can decorate their homes with beautiful flowers. Each of us is a cracked pot in one way or another, but there is still no limit to the beauty we can create."

From that day on, the cracked pot knew just how wonderful it really was.

—TRADITIONAL STORY FROM INDIA ADAPTED
BY DAN GIBSON, ©1999, *WWW.DANGIBSON.NET*

week 3:
Journal

I never know what I think about something until I read what I've written on it.

—WILLIAM FAULKNER

Journaling is a powerful technique that opens the door to you:

- To what you think
- To who you are
- To your inner wisdom
- To guide you through the murk and mire of overwhelming emotions and dramas
- To illuminate the path from darkness right (write!) into the light

Journaling can be done with a question or topic in mind, as a way to record your day, or as stream-of-consciousness, by putting pen to paper and writing whatever comes to mind. Whether journaling is a new technique for you, or if you have been journal writing since you got your first diary as a child that came with a lock and key and the word DIARY written in gold letters, journal writing provides a direct path to peace and happiness.

There have been times in my life that my journal has been my best friend, accepting all I write with no judgments, always available. After spending time with my journal I feel renewed and refreshed. I began writing in a diary when I was a child. My journals take up a couple of shelves on a bookcase. They are all sizes, shapes, and fabrics, handmade by artists or factory-made and mass-produced. I have drawn in them, written in them, used special pens, and been a poet in them. I have written my secret thoughts and my heart's desires. I have written how others have been mean to me and how I have been cruel to others. I have made lists of plans. For many years when I was single I wrote a journal that was a call to the universe for my mate. I envisioned I would give this beautiful flowered book to him when we married. Years later I gave it to him on our wedding night. Well, I'm single again—and I've written another journal as a call to my soulmate for the next chapter of my life!

Recently I read many of my journals and noticed how often I repeated dramas in which I was not enough: not pretty enough, not smart enough, not sexy enough, not loveable enough, not good enough, not thin enough, not wealthy enough. Those old stories are no longer the central theme in my life. It may be time to burn or bury these journals, since my story of peace and happiness now takes center stage.

On March 17, 2003, I burned my journals—and they served me, yet again, as my old story transformed into ashes that I used as fertilizer in my garden to nourish new blooms.

Enjoy journaling this week and notice the impact of writing (righting) in your life when you journal as a daily practice.

HOW TO DO IT

DAY 1: If you have a journal, use it; if you don't, get one. It can be a special book you love seeing and touching or simply a spiral notebook. You may get a special pen you love or use any one that is nearby. Journal writing is a pathway to an intimate relationship with yourself, so honor this relationship.

Write for ten minutes, anything that comes to your mind, even if what comes to your mind is, *"I don't know what to write."* Simply write for ten minutes. If you are stumped about how to start you can start by writing: *"Today I am writing in my journal for ten minutes."*

DAY 2: Write in your journal for fifteen minutes today about your heart's desire. Title your page My Heart's Desire and write. You may notice, when you look at it after you have finished writing for fifteen minutes, that there is variation in your handwriting in different parts of what you have written. I have noticed that my handwriting is very much influenced by what I am feeling. Often during one session of writing I feel many feelings that are reflected in my handwriting. This is one of the reasons I prefer to journal-write by hand rather than on a computer.

DAY 3: Choose a topic, issue, or question you are concerned about and write about it for fifteen minutes. Some possibilities are:

· My ideal job
· How can I be loving with my family?
· What are the beliefs of someone who experiences abundance?
· How can I experience greater well-being in my life?
· How can I see my financial crisis through the eyes of love?

Remember that at any point while you are writing if you hear a voice in your mind saying, *"I don't know what else to write about this,"* write that down. Write whatever pops into your mind. This is not about creating a literary masterpiece. It is about you communicating with you.

DAY 4: Any time during the day when you are feeling off-center, anxious, worried, or disconnected, stop what you are doing as soon as you can and write what you are feeling. Allow whatever words come to your mind out through your pen. Write until you are feeling all right again. This is a powerful way to acknowledge what you are feeling and to move on from there. When we resist feeling what we feel, the feeling persists either in our consciousness or below the surface of our awareness and continues to influence our perception of the world. When we allow what we are feeling and acknowledge it, we are able to move through it and move on.

DAY 5: Write your personal history from the point of view of being enough: good enough, smart enough, handsome enough, beautiful enough, athletic enough, sexy enough, loveable enough. For some of us this is a stretch, because the dramas and traumas of our lives have been the main themes of our personal histories. So if you were in an abusive family, rather than focusing on that, remember your next-door neighbor who always had a kind word for you. You now have the opportunity to free yourself from an old story that no longer serves you and to write a new one. You may be surprised, as you get into this journaling exercise, at the buried happy memories that pop up. Do this for at least fifteen minutes.

DAY 6: Choose any topic or simply follow your stream of consciousness and journal for about fifteen minutes.

DAY 7: Write your reflections on journaling.

- What was your experience journaling?
- How did you feel after writing each day?
- Did you prefer a having a specific topic or stream-of-consciousness or a combination of both?
- How did journaling contribute to you being peace and happiness?

Writing crystallizes thought and thought produces action.

—PAUL J. MEYER

week 4:
Be Grateful

If the only prayer you ever say in your life is, "Thank You,"
it will be enough.

—Meister Eckhart

Being grateful acknowledges what we have attracted into our lives. People seem to have more practice noticing what isn't working and what is lacking in their lives than the abundant gifts in their world. This is a learned habit. Practicing gratitude and appreciation creates a new pattern in our thoughts and behaviors. With this practice, we see the world from a new point of view. It requires practice to strengthen your perception of gratitude. The practice begins with your intent to nurture this viewpoint and your conscious awareness to notice where you put your attention. If you notice your attention is on lack, acknowledge yourself for noticing and then focus your attention on what is abundant in your life, what you are grateful for. If you notice your consciousness is focused on gratitude, give yourself a pat on the back to reinforce the strengthening of an attitude of gratitude in your life.

HOW TO DO IT

DAY 1: When you wake up in the morning, express your gratitude for the gift of the new day, and before you go to sleep at night, express your appreciation for the day you've lived.

DAY 2: Once an hour, stop what you are doing and focus on what you are grateful for.

DAY 3: Before you go to sleep, write down five things you are grateful for on that day: for example, I am grateful for my health, I am grateful for my family, I am grateful I flossed my teeth, I am grateful for my eyesight, I am grateful for the sun rising this morning, I am grateful I meditated for twenty minutes, and so forth. This is a powerful daily practice. Do it every day for a month and notice the shift in perception you experience having strengthened your muscle of appreciation. Continue doing it every day.

DAY 4: Find inspiring quotes about gratitude and put them on your refrigerator. Enter them as reminders in your Palm Pilot, on your calendar, and on your screen saver. When you notice them, stop for a moment and express and experience your gratitude for the life you have and the people in it.

DAY 5: Express your gratitude throughout the day by saying, "Thank you." Set a challenge for yourself. Today, I am saying thank you fifty times, one hundred times, or even more! Remember, you may say thank you to the person in the car in front of you who is driving slowly for giving you an opportunity to practice patience. See if you can find at least one thing to be thankful for in every situation you are in today.

DAY 6: Begin a daily practice of identifying one thing each day for which you have never before expressed your appreciation. For instance:

- I am grateful my toenails grow.
- I am grateful for the wrinkly lines on my fingers that make it easy for me to bend my fingers.
- I am grateful for the parents of the person at the checkout counter of the supermarket who smiled at me today while checking out my groceries.
- I am grateful for hearing the cell phone calls of people who died on 9/11 reminding me that love is the greatest gift we have to give.

DAY 7: Write your reflections on being grateful.

- How did focusing on what you are grateful for impact your peace and happiness?
- How can you incorporate being grateful into your daily life? Do it.

Both abundance and lack exist simultaneously in our lives, as parallel realities. It is always our conscious choice which secret garden we will tend. When we choose not to focus on what is missing from our lives but are grateful for the abundance that's present—love, health, family, friends, work, the joys of nature and personal pursuits that bring us pleasure, the wasteland of illusion falls away and we experience Heaven on Earth.

—SARAH BAN BREATHNACH, *SIMPLE ABUNDANCE*

week 5:
Use the Creative Power of Your Word

The word is not just a sound or a written symbol. The word is a force; it is the power you have to express and communicate, to think, and thereby to create the events of your life.

—DON MIGUEL RUIZ

Honoring the creative power of your word, what you say and what you think, is the foundation for the experience you create in your life. The first words of the Bible are, "In the beginning was the word, and the word was with God, and the word was God." In the bestseller, *The Four Agreements*, don Miguel Ruiz describes four agreements to live by in order to experience heaven on earth. The first and most important agreement is being impeccable with your word. At first, I thought this simply meant that if I say I will meet you at 5:00 P.M., then I make sure to keep that agreement. If for some reason that is not possible, I'll do my best to let you know. While this is important, the deeper meaning of being impeccable with your word is to think and say loving and accepting words about yourself and others. Most of the time we are asleep to the words we say and the tape that runs in our mind as self-talk.

For example, have you heard yourself say, "I am so stupid," or "I never do anything right," or "My husband/wife is such an idiot." As you read this, you might be thinking, "Yeah, I've said those things, what's the big deal?" The big deal is that what we believe, expressed in our thoughts and words, is the experience we create. Keep in mind that beliefs are simply habitual thoughts that we have come to consider truth. Our thoughts create our reality. Our thoughts are the operating system of the life we create and live. If you want to see what you are thinking, look at the life you are living. It is the external manifestation of the thoughts you have had. Are you experiencing peace and happiness? If yes, consciously continue with the kind of thoughts you are having. If no, wake up to what you think and what you say, and think thoughts and say words that support your peace and happiness now.

HOW TO DO IT

Sit in silence each day and listen to your thoughts. Consciously change them when they are not supportive of peace and happiness. Start with five minutes per day and extend the length of time (to thirty minutes per day; twenty minutes twice per day; five minutes every hour; experiment).

DAY 1: Make a list of statements you can say to yourself that are kind, respectful, and loving. Some examples are:

- I have a great sense of humor.
- I am loving.
- I am a great friend.
- I am reliable.
- I am a great chef.

Choose one of these statements each day and first thing in the morning and just before you go to sleep, say it to yourself while looking in the mirror. You can also write the statement on a Post-It note and carry it with you during the day to remind you to repeat the words once every hour.

DAY 2: Make a list of the statements you think and say about yourself and others that are abusive and judgmental. When you hear yourself say or think these thoughts, change the language of your thoughts at that moment. It is crucial that you not judge and criticize yourself, as it's another form of self-abuse. When you notice abusive thoughts and words, acknowledge yourself for being awake and aware and have a new thought. With this increased awareness, you can make conscious choices about what you think and say.

DAY 3: Use your feelings as a guidance system. When you are feeling peace and happiness, notice the thoughts you are thinking; when you are feeling angry, unhappy, sad, frustrated, alone, or afraid, notice what you believe at the moment. Remember it is not bad that you are having these feelings. We have the power to change our thoughts and thereby our points of view and beliefs.

DAY 4: Make direct statements (for example, "I'd like to go to the movies, and I'd like you to join me," rather than "What do you want to do?"). Often we know exactly what we want if we get quiet and focused enough to listen rather than hiding what we want in questions and vague statements.

DAY 5: Keep your word and honor your agreements. Notice the agreements you make with yourself and honor them; listen to the commitments you make with others and keep them. When you make changes in these agreements, allow your words to reflect your integrity. Two months ago I told someone that I planned to attend a course he was teaching. In the intervening weeks I changed my work schedule and could no longer attend his course. I left him a phone message. As I was beginning to write this chapter he called and asked me about the course. I told him it didn't work for me to take it right then. He said that if it didn't work we could discuss being flexible with the schedule. I continued to say that it didn't work for me, and he asked, "Is it that you prefer not to take it now or is it that the schedule doesn't work for you?" The truth was that I preferred not to take the course now. I thanked him for his coaching. Honoring my word is saying what I mean!

DAY 6: Put reminders around your home and workplace to honor the creative power of your word. For example:

· Thoughts are real things.
· Honor the creative power of your word.
· Eliminate gossip.
· Think love.
· Speak love.
· My experience begins with my word.

DAY 7: Write what you have learned about the creative power of your word.

· What did you notice this week when you focused on your word?
· What are your challenges in being conscious of your thoughts and words?
· What helps you to use the creative power of your word to expand your peace and happiness?

You can measure the impeccability of your word by your level of self-love. How much you love yourself and how you feel about yourself are directly proportionate to the quality and integrity of your word.

—DON MIGUEL RUIZ

week 6:
Breathe

Breathe-in experience, breathe-out poetry.
—MURIEL RUKEYSER

Breathe. Breath is life. Focusing on your breath is the most powerful natural resource you have for stepping into peace and happiness. Right now, stop for a moment and focus on your breath. Close your eyes and focus your attention on your in-breath and your out-breath. Do this five times. What do you notice? Are you more aware of your body? Are you feeling quieter? I notice that when I focus my attention on my breath, actually following the path of my breath as it enters my body through my nose, circulates throughout my body, and leaves my body through my mouth, I feel a deeper sense of relaxation and calm, more fully present in the moment. This is the power of focusing on your breath. Focus on breath is also the foundation of Buddhist meditation exercises, breath work used in rebirthing, bioenergetic therapy practices and childbirth exercises. This week, breathe consciously. Any time you notice yourself experiencing undue stress or tension, or you are rushing around and have lost connection with being in the present moment, focus your attention on your breath. B R E A T H E. Consider these possibilities:

- With each inhalation God, or Source Energy, is breathing into you, giving to you, and with each exhalation you are giving your unique contribution to Source Energy.
- We are connected with all beings, all that is, through our breath. We are inhaling one another's exhalations all the time. While it looks as if we are separated from one another by the space between our bodies and the objects of our world, we are actually connected through our breath.
- As breath enters our body, it is charged with the vibration and frequency of the thoughts we are thinking. As we exhale, we are exhaling both air and the emotional charge, the vibration, of the thought that is being exhaled at that moment. We spread an emotional frequency through our breath. With this in mind, thoughts are real things, and

what we think, therefore, makes a very big impact in the world. We pass our thoughts around through our breath! What do you contribute to the world through you exhalations? Love, fear, happiness, anxiety, heaven, or hell?

HOW TO DO IT

DAY 1: Become aware of your breath. Put a B R E AT H E screen saver on your computer. Put Post-It notes around your house, workplace, and car to remind you to B R E A T H E. When you see these reminders, stop and B R E AT H E. Take full, deep breaths, using your diaphragm, so that when you inhale your belly expands and when you exhale your belly contracts. Experiment: focus simply on expanding and contracting your diaphragm, and notice how breath is automatically drawn into your body and expelled from your body. Play with having your breath breathe you. Do a search on the internet, in your local library or bookstore, and ask a yoga teacher to give you suggestions for different breathing exercises.

DAY 2: Meditate for twenty minutes, focusing your attention on your breath. When your mind wanders, bring your attention back to your inhalation and your exhalation. You can do this in one sitting or two sittings of ten minutes each.

DAY 3: Meditate for twenty minutes and focus on moving your breath through your entire body. Start at your feet and inhale into your feet. Feel your feet relax as you exhale. To use your breath to enhance your body awareness even more, you can focus on one toe at a time, one finger at a time, and so forth. After each exhalation move your attention and breath up your body, starting with your toes, your ankles, your calves, your knees, moving up your body to include your liver, your heart, your ears, your eyelids, your lips, and so forth.

DAY 4: Any time you feel tension in your body, breathe into that part of your body, and as you exhale, allow the tension to leave your body and breathe it into the earth. The earth has the powerful ability to take whatever is given to her and transform it into support and nourishment. You can use this exercise with worrisome and fearful thoughts as well.

DAY 5: Once an hour, for five consecutive inhalations, imagine that God, Source Energy, the loving energy of the universe, is breathing, gently blowing breath into your being. Each exhalation is your gift to Source Energy. I play with this on my morning walks on the beach. When the wind is blowing, I stand with my mouth open and allow the air to fill my body, and then, as I exhale, I give to the wind the air that is moving through my being. I have a very vivid memory of doing this at 8:15 A.M. the morning of September 11, 2001. The beach was spectacular on that crystal-clear day. The tide was roaring, and the wind was blowing. I walked to the jetty and stood, facing the ocean. The wind embraced me, and the sound of the waves were crescendos. I thought, "This is power. This is the kind of power that is present in the universe. Fill me." I opened my mouth and allowed the air to fill my being. I exhaled and added my breath to the wind. A short time later, planes crashed into the World Trade Center, the Pentagon, and a field in Pennsylvania. Did the air already carry the power that was being unleashed that day?

DAY 6: Meditate for twenty minutes on the words of Thich Nhat Hanh, a Buddhist monk, contemporary meditation teacher, and author:

> Breathing in I calm my mind and body.
> Breathing out I smile.
> Breathing in I dwell in the moment.
> This is the only moment.

DAY 7: Write about what you have learned this week by focusing your attention on your breath.

- How did this focus on your breath contribute to your peace and happiness?
- What is your most powerful insight about your breath?
- How can you use your breath on a daily basis to experience greater peace and happiness?

week 7:
Use Virtual Reality

In your virtual reality, make it as you want it to be.

—ABRAHAM

Using virtual reality involves tapping into the full resources of our imagination to create a reality that supports our highest well-being. This is also known as creative visualization. One of the fascinating aspects of being human is that what we focus our attention on results in the experience we have. We don't actually have to be in a situation to experience its impact. We can simply imagine it, create a virtual reality of a circumstance with the full resources of our imagination, and it is as if we are having the experience. For example, you are on vacation, lounging on a comfortable chair near the water's edge. You hear the sound of the turquoise surf lapping against the shore. You smell the gentle hint of salt in the air. You feel the warmth of the sun combined with a gentle breeze caressing your body. You turn your head slightly to the right and see your lover in the chair at your side. Notice how you feel now, having just read this beach scene virtual reality.

Suddenly, the thought of the pressures and demands of home and work enters your mind and hooks your attention. Immediately you feel tightness in your shoulders, butterflies in your stomach, and the words in your mind sound something like, "Oh, no, I don't want to go back to work." A feeling of dissatisfaction and unhappiness fills your being. Even though you are still on the beach and your physical environment has remained pleasurable, your focus in a different virtual reality changed your experience. When we realize the profound life-changing power we have available to us at each moment simply by where we direct our attention, we can experience peace and happiness every day.

Most of us have learned to focus on lack in our lives. When we are happy, we expect that it won't last long, or something will happen to ruin it. Using virtual reality to create pleasurable experiences is very helpful in creating new patterns of thought, focusing on abundance, love, heaven, and peace and happiness. When experiences of lack, fear, hell, and suffering hook our attention, we can acknowledge them and with greater ease move through them and choose peace and happiness once again.

Note it is crucial that you not judge yourself when fear, anger, lack, and hell take center stage in your life. Here are some things to keep in mind when this does occur:

- Old patterns operate on automatic, and it takes attention and discipline to create new patterns of thought and behavior.
- Fear, anger, lack, and hell are powerful calls for love in our life. It is not bad that we are feeling them. It is a reminder that we are out of touch with Source Energy, the loving energy of the universe. Rather than getting seduced by the drama of the situation, the best place to focus our attention is on changing our vibration, getting centered, connecting with Source Energy.

Using virtual reality allows us to practice having good-feeling thoughts and to become proficient at changing our experience in the moment. It can also be used to envision your heart's desire and to *see* your highest image for well-being in every situation you are stepping into. This week you will consciously hone your expertise as a virtual reality creator. Remember, the only limits are those you allow, so be peace and happiness each step of the way.

HOW TO DO IT

DAY 1: Make a pleasure list. This is a list of things you can use to create a virtual reality. Choose one item on your list and once an hour for thirty seconds create a virtual reality of it by:

- Closing your eyes and being there.
- Putting yourself into the scene. Be specific; include where you are, time of day, what you are wearing, and so forth.
- Experiencing your virtual reality with all your senses. What are you hearing, seeing, touching, tasting, and feeling?

Any time during the thirty seconds you feel anything other than pleasure, get out of the virtual reality and start again. It may be helpful to start with scenes that don't involve other people, since we have a tendency to bring others into our virtual reality whom we want to change and fix. The purpose of this exercise is to give us practice feeling good, *not* to fix people or circumstances in our lives.

DAY 2: Once an hour, repeat Day 1 with the same or different pleasure list items.

DAY 3: Repeat Day 1. During the day, whenever you notice you are flirting with or are in hell, create a pleasurable thirty-second virtual reality. You may be able to unhook energetically after thirty seconds, or you may have to play with virtual reality repeatedly. Remember, this is a practice in changing your focus and thereby your experience in the moment. Once you are in a more centered space, you will be more open and able to move through whatever circumstances are present.

DAY 4: Repeat Day 1, and five times today do a virtual reality of your heart's desire for thirty seconds. See your heart's desire as accomplished. Savor it, taste it, feel it, and know that the universe is saying a resounding, YES.

DAY 5: Use virtual reality to *see* every situation you are stepping into as fully and completely satisfying. For instance, as you are getting out of bed in the morning, see yourself stepping out of the shower feeling refreshed, alert, clean, and eager for a satisfying day. As you get ready to leave the house in the morning see yourself arriving at your destination safely and having enjoyed the journey. Play with this, have fun, and enjoy your day.

DAY 6: Practice using virtual reality throughout the day, once an hour, and whenever you want to transform hell to heaven. Strengthen your new habit of tapping into virtual reality to uplift your experience and set your direction.

DAY 7: Continue using virtual reality and write your reflections on consciously using virtual reality this week.

- What did you learn?
- What was most surprising to you?
- How can you keep this muscle strong and toned? Do it.

WEEK 8:
Be Kind

This is my simple religion. There is no need for temples; no need for complicated philosophy. Our own brain, our own heart is our temple; the philosophy is kindness.

—THE DALAI LAMA

Being kind to ourselves and to everyone in the world doesn't require great wealth, large chunks of time, or a complicated procedure to follow. Kindness manifests itself in the way you care for and love yourself and others. It is a point of view, the glasses through which we view the world. Kindness is expressed in our thoughts, words, and actions. Being kind can be as simple as saying "thank you" to the cashier at your local supermarket after you have paid for your groceries, traveling far to be with a friend in need, paying the toll for the car behind you, or saying a prayer for people involved in a news story of suffering you just read. Being kind is how we apply the Golden Rule—do unto others as you would have others do unto you. In all the religions of the world, there is a version of the Golden Rule, also known as the ethic of reciprocity. Our personal experience of peace and happiness depends on being kind. The possibility of peace in our families, workplaces, communities, and institutions in the world requires that we be kind to one another and remember that we are all connected and what is done to any part effects the whole.

Kindness has a ripple effect often greater than the act itself. The receiver is happy, surprised, and often wakes up to the present moment. When recipients of the kindness tell their stories to others, the kindness extends outward and seeds the idea of being kind in those who hear about it. Imagine a world where spontaneous acts of kindness are a given. Often the biggest receiver is the one who has performed the act, as the energy of lovingkindness moves through you as you express kindness. This week, to deepen your peace and happiness, be kind. When you get a prompting to offer a helping hand, do it; if you notice you are feeling a bit shy and embarrassed about doing a good deed, do it anyway. New patterns of behavior usually feel awkward at first.

HOW TO DO IT

DAY 1: Be kind to yourself today in your thoughts, words, and actions. Any time you notice you are being critical or judgmental of yourself in your thoughts or words, change those thoughts and words. If you have a deadline to meet at work and one of your coworkers has stopped by to shoot the breeze, be kind to yourself by gently asserting yourself and saying you have work to do and will have to cut the conversation short. Treat yourself as though you are precious, because you are.

DAY 2: Make a kindness list to be aware of the various faces of kindness. Here are some ideas to start your list:

- Help someone carry their groceries.
- Pay the toll for the car behind you.
- Call a family member or friend and tell them how special they are to you.
- Anonymously leave chocolate kisses on the desk of your coworkers.
- Leave a thank-you note for your mail carrier.
- Donate a pint of blood.
- Drop some loose change on the street for someone to find.
- Put money into a parking meter whose time has expired.

DAY 3: Be kind. Do one act of kindness for everyone you are with today. A smile and a "thank you" can go a long way. Thoughts are real things, and we can express our kindness through our thoughts. Often when I am waiting for a bus, I will send one of the following thoughts to everyone who passes in front of me, and in New York City, that's a lot of people!

- God loves you.
- You are love.
- You live in a loving world.

When I do this, I always experience peace and happiness, and my world is richer, because I take a moment to actually see the people who are passing directly through my world.

DAY 4: Read the book and/or see the movie, *Pay It Forward*, and then pay it forward. *Pay It Forward* is an inspiring story of a twelve-year-old boy's plan to change the world for the better. His idea is that when someone does a favor for you, you "pay it forward" by doing a favor or act of kindness for three other people. As each person who has received a favor "pays it forward" to three other people, a chain of human kindness is quickly achieved.

DAY 5: Customize your screen saver and put Post-It notes around your house and workplace with kindness reminder quotes. Here are some to choose from, and be creative and make up your own:

- Remember there's no such thing as a small act of kindness. Every act creates a ripple with no logical end.—Scott Adams
- Forget injuries, never forget kindnesses.—Aesop
- No act of kindness, however small, is ever wasted.—Aesop
- Little deeds of kindness, little words of love, help to make earth happy like the heaven above.—Julia A. Fletcher Carney
- I am kind.

DAY 6: Talk with five people today about the power of being kind.

DAY 7: Write your reflections on being kind.

- What did you learn this week by consciously being kind?
- How can you incorporate kindness into your daily life? Do it.

Just because an animal is large, it doesn't mean he doesn't want kindness; however big Tigger seems to be, remember that he wants as much kindness as Roo.

—*POOH'S LITTLE INSTRUCTION BOOK*,
INSPIRED BY A. A. MILNE

Being Kind

Monday afternoon, Labor Day, 1999. It was a beautiful summer afternoon. I was driving in my fire-engine red Miata convertible, with my gray-and-white sheepdog, Rosie, in the passenger seat, moving at sixty-five miles per hour. As I slowed down, approaching the tollbooth, I had to move into the long cash line to pay my toll, since I didn't have an E-Z Pass on my car. I was moving at a snail's pace. As I sat there, holding Rosie with my right hand and my toll in my left hand, I heard that still small voice within say, "Pay the toll for the people behind you." I thought, "I don't know if I want to do that. Well, it would be a random act of kindness. It would be a nice thing to do."

33

I started feeling embarrassed about doing this random act of kind-ness. What would the people behind me think? What would the toll-taker think? Then I thought, "What does it matter what they think?" I had made a commitment to listen to and follow the instructions of that still small voice within. So, continuing to hold Rosie, I reached into my wallet and got more money, preparing to pay the toll for the car behind me.

There were still about seven cars in front of me, so I started watching my rearview mirror to see the people in the car behind me. I began to fantasize about what their reaction would be when they drove to the tollbooth and the attendant told them that their toll had already been paid. There was a man, woman, and child in the car. I thought they would be happy. I imagined their smiles while telling their family and friends about discovering, as they drove through the tollbooth, that their toll had already been paid. So I was feeling quite good about this act of kindness I was ready to perform, when all of a sudden, on my right, a pickup truck started cutting in front of me. Instantly I was transformed. "What did this guy think he was doing cutting in front of me? I was in line in front of him!" I held fast to my position, not letting that big pickup truck edge me in my little Miata out. "I'll show him."

Well, in the midst of showing him, it wound up that the pickup truck became the car behind me! What was I going to do now, faced with this enormous dilemma? Do I still pay the toll for the car behind me? Do I reinforce his behavior of attempting to cut me off? Through my irritated chatter I again heard that still small voice within saying calmly and clearly, "Pay the toll for the car behind you. Pay the toll for the car behind you." As I went through the tollbooth I paid my toll and the toll for the car behind me.

As I write this story I'm reminded that oftentimes I want to nego-tiate with God, and with God's wisdom within me. I want to decide whom I'll be kind to. The challenge, for me, is simply to listen to and follow the instructions of that still, small voice within when I am prompted to be kind.

—SR

week 9:
Pamper Yourself

If not now, when?
If not you, who?

—SR

Pampering yourself is a requirement for peace and happiness. Sometimes there are prerequisites for courses you want to enroll in; pampering yourself is a prerequisite for peace and happiness. Many of us mean to do it, like to do it, want to do it, but when our schedules get busy or our finances are stretched, pampering ourselves falls by the wayside, just when we need it the most. While pampering can be costly and time-consuming, it doesn't have to be. If you have a bathtub and running water, you can create a spa experience in your bathroom. If you have a tape or CD player, or a radio, you can surround yourself with music that soothes your soul, calms your mind, and lifts your spirit. And yes, you can go to a spa for a week surrounded by the healing embrace of nature, get daily massages, take naps, stretch your body, take some cardio-pumping hikes, and practice meditation to pamper yourself as well. Your biggest block to pampering yourself is usually you and your habit of putting yourself last on your to-do list. This week you are number one, and when you complete this prerequisite, notice peace and happiness popping up more regularly in your life.

HOW TO DO IT

resources

- ~ *2,001 Ways to Pamper Yourself* by Lorraine Bodger, Kansas City: Andrews McMeel, 1999.
- ~ *Simple Indulgence: Easy, Everyday Things to Do for Me* by Janet Eastman, Kansas City: Andrews McMeel, 1999.
- ~ *50 Simple Ways to Pamper Yourself* by Stephanie L. Tourles, Pownal, VT: Storey Books, 1999.

DAYS 1-7: Make a list of ways to pamper yourself and choose one for each day and do it; I repeat, Do It, DO IT. Here are some ideas to start your list:

- Get a massage.
- Trade foot massages with a family member or friend.
- Take a bubble bath.
- Go to the barber and get a hot shaving cream shave.
- Get a manicure and pedicure.
- Go for a walk.
- Listen to great music.
- Get a custom-made shirt.
- Get a golf lesson.
- Write in your journal (This is a good one to choose for Day 7).
- Put a "Do Not Disturb" sign on your office or bedroom door.
- Make love.
- Read a novel.
- Curl up and watch a movie.
- Take a nap.
- Meditate.
- Have a cup of tea with a friend.
- Use the good dishes.
- Take a spa vacation.
- Arrange a phone date with a dear friend.
- Spend an afternoon at the movies.

I pampered myself today by: _____.

Note: The above statement is purposefully written in the past tense. Complete it in the morning as though you have already pampered yourself. Writing in the past tense is a powerful mind game that gives legs to your intention to pamper yourself. I often write items on my to-do list in the past tense. I then feel more energized, as though they are done!

DAY 2: I pampered myself today by: _____.

DAY 3: I pampered myself today by: _____.

DAY 4: I pampered myself today by: _____.

DAY 5: I pampered myself today by: _____.

DAY 6: I pampered myself today by: _____.

DAY 7: I pampered myself today by: _____.

Write your reflections of pampering yourself:

- What did you notice by consciously pampering yourself each day?
- Make a daily pampering appointment with yourself for each day for the rest of your life! Get out your appointment book or your Palm Pilot and write them down.

week 10:
Read Inspiring Words

Quotes influence and move us. Once we hear those words and feel the impact, they forever help shape our thinking. Words are the language of the mind; we do not give enough importance to their ability to hurt or heal.

—DAVID BROMFIELD

Reading inspiring words is a powerful way to focus your attention. Being peace and happiness begins, as all experiences begin, with a thought charged with an energetic vibration/frequency (energy in motion – e-motion = emotion). Therefore inspiring words, in the form of a single word, one-line quotes, poetry, essays, and stories, have the power to focus your attention in the moment, awakening and reinforcing your experience of peace and happiness. Words and sounds have the power to transform your experience: soothe a broken heart, put a smile on your face, offer a new view of a situation, and evoke the sacred that is always present in the moment. Read inspiring words aloud this week; feel each word resonate within your being. As you read, if your attention wanders, go back to the beginning of what you are reading with the intent of being in communion (common union) with the words, allowing them to illuminate your way and your day.

HOW TO DO IT

Begin and end each day this week with an inspirational reading. This may be a continuation of readings from a book of daily readings that you are already familiar with, or you may choose a particular poet to read each morning, or scan the books in your home and notice which one *feels* just right for this assignment. Focus your full attention on your reading. Put down your coffee cup and clear your mind of everything but the present moment and the gifts of inspiration in the words you are reading aloud. I often do this reading in bed, upon waking up, and before going to sleep. If you have an altar in your home or a special room or chair you may want to read there.

Some books of daily readings that have inspired me are:

38

- *Simple Abundance* by Sarah Ban Breathnach, New York: Warner Books, 1995.
- *The Seven Spiritual Laws of Success* by Deepak Chopra, San Rafael, CA: Amber-Allen Books, 1995.
- *The Courage to Change* by Al-Anon Family Groups, Virginia Beach: Al-Anon Family Headquarters, 1992.
- *One Day My Soul Just Opened Up* by Iyanla Vanzant, New York: Simon and Schuster, 1998.
- *A Course in Miracles* by The Foundation for Inner Peace, New York: Viking, 1996.
- *Sacred Intentions: Daily Inspiration to Strengthen the Spirit* by Rabbi Kerry M. Olitzky and Rabbi Lori Forman, Woodstock, VT: Jewish Lights Publishing, 1999.
- *The Promise of a New Day* by Karen Casey and Martha Vanceburg, San Francisco: HarperSanFrancisco, 1996.
- *Night Light: A Book of Nighttime Meditations* by Amy E. Dean, Center City, MN: Hazelden, 1996.
- Mark Rosenbush's website: *http://upi.cc/peace_begins/*.

DAY 1: Search the Web for inspiring quotes. Simply type "inspiring quotes" into your browser or choose a specific topic and type: "faith quotes," or "love quotes," or "peace and happiness quotes," and so forth. Choose a few to write down and post them where they will capture your attention: on your screen saver, in your appointment book, as a message on your Palm Pilot, on your bathroom mirror, on your dashboard, on your closet door, on your bedside table, and so forth. When you see them, stop what you are doing for a moment, read them, and invite the words to fill your being. Listen to and read "Interview with God" on the following website: *http://168.143.173.209.* Explore the *Beliefnet.com* website.

DAY 2: Read "The Prayer for Peace & Happiness" on page 3 once an hour. At the end of the day, write about the impact of saying and focusing on this prayer once per hour.

DAY 3: Go to your local library, bookstore, or to your own or a friend's bookcase and choose a book with words of inspiration to read and begin reading it. If you are like me, you may have books in your personal library that you bought and have never looked at. This may be the time to open one of them.

DAY 4: Begin an inspiration journal. This will be your personal book of inspiration. Begin today to write quotes in it, adding to it whenever you come across something that deepens your experience of peace and happiness. While you can do this on your computer in a file entitled "Inspiration Journal," I have found that the act of writing and saying the words aloud as I form them seems to amplify my experience. Experiment.

DAY 5: Write your own words of inspiration. This may be a poem or a response to any or all of the following questions:

· The key to peace and happiness is:_____.
· The greatest life lesson is:_____.
· The most important words of wisdom I want to share with the children in my life are:_____.

DAY 6: Share inspiring words that are meaningful and powerful for you with three people.

DAY 7: Write about your experience of reading inspiring words.

· How did this effect your day?
· If this is a new practice for you, do you want to continue it daily?
· Is there a particular prayer or words that you want to focus on regularly as a way to direct your attention when you are stressed and off-center?

Come

Come, whoever you are! Wanderer, worshipper, Lover of Leaving
Come.
This is not a caravan of despair. It doesn't matter if you've
broken your vow a thousand times, still
Come,
and yet again
Come!

—RUMI

week 11:
Eliminate Gossip

*Gossip is black magic at its very worst because it is pure
poison. We learned how to gossip by agreement. When we were
children, we heard the adults around us gossiping all the
time, openly giving their opinions about other people. They
even had opinions about people they didn't know. Emotional
poison was transferred along with the opinions, and we
learned this as the normal way to communicate.*

—DON MIGUEL RUIZ

Eliminating gossip is one way we honor the creative power of our word and support our search for peace and happiness. Gossip is a form of judgment and abuse, either about ourselves or others. While the intent is not always malicious, it is the telling and retelling of a story that gets embellished in the telling and charged with emotional fuel that reinforces drama. Remember, our words have creative power: what we think and say, charged with emotions, is what we create. Gossip is like casting a spell, feeding a story of woe, and reinforcing the exact behavior that annoys us to begin with. If you feel yourself eager to spread the news about what you heard about so-and-so, or if you are in search of someone to tell the continuing drama of your life, just don't do it! At first, this might feel uncomfortable, since so much of our communication is about our opinions of others or about some continuing saga in our own lives. Some of us, like me, who have had talk therapy, have become so adept at *sharing* our story that when we eliminate gossip, we are initially at a loss about what to say to others. Keep in mind that silence is okay, even though we may not be used to it. Commenting on the present moment, the sound of the wind, the fragrance of honeysuckle in the air, the moon, the taste of the food we are eating is okay conversation. Eliminate gossip this week, and if you find yourself seduced and eager to get into the muck and mire of a juicy story, with many twists and turns in the plot, take a deep breath and choose, in the moment, to eliminate gossip.

HOW TO DO IT

DAY 1: Think before you speak. If it's gossip, don't say it. If you're not sure whether or not it is gossip, don't say it.

DAY 2: Notice when you do gossip and stop or change the direction of the conversation.

DAY 3: When you are with others who are gossiping practice saying, "I'd prefer not gossiping about _____," or "Rather than gossiping about _____, lets talk about what's working in our lives," or "I'm practicing not gossiping and fueling the drama in my life—would you help me by changing the subject?" Or simply, and this is often the easiest, change the subject.

DAY 4: Share good news about what is going on in your life.

DAY 5: Notice how often the conversations you are involved in are based on gossip. The more you become aware of this, the more you can change the course of a conversation midstream or simply remove yourself from it. Make sure you do not go on a crusade and judge others. Simply practice eliminating gossip and notice how that impacts those around you.

DAY 6: Share with five people what you have learned about yourself by eliminating gossip this week.

DAY 7: Write your reflections on eliminating gossip.

- What did you learn about yourself?
- What made it hard to eliminate gossip; what made it easy?
- How do you plan to continue eliminating gossip in your life?

The Monk and the Peasant

A peasant once unthinkingly spread tales about a friend.
But later found the rumors false and hoped to make amend.
He sought the counsel of a monk, a man esteemed and wise,
Who heard the peasant's story through and felt he must advise.
The kind monk said: "If you would have a mind again at peace,
I have a plan whereby you may from trouble find release.
Go fill a bag with chicken down and to each dooryard go
And lay one fluffy feather where the streams of gossip show."
The peasant did as he was told and to the monk returned,
Elated that his penance was a thing so quickly earned.
"Not yet," the old monk sternly said, "Take up your bag once
    more
And gather up the feathers that you placed at every door."
The peasant, eager to atone, went hastening to obey,
No feathers met his sight, the wind had blown them all away.

—MARGARET E. BRUNER

week 12:
Forgive

Forgiveness is the answer to the child's dream of a miracle by which what is broken is made whole again, what is soiled is made clean.

—Dag Hammarskjöld

To forgive requires a shift in consciousness and perception that opens up space in your heart where you are imprisoned by guilt, blame, shame, anger, and regret. Whether we are forgiving ourselves, someone else, a group, or an institution, the forgiver receives the greatest gift. An interesting thing about human beings is that we seem to be the only species that continually punishes itself by reliving situations from the past. Whether we regret something we have said or done or blame someone else for what he or she has said or didn't say or has done to us, each time we remember the situation we reactivate the feelings of hurt, pain, anger, and sadness. Forgiveness is the action that releases and frees us from past pain, opening our heart and mind to love—being peace and happiness.

HOW TO DO IT

DAY 1: Make a forgiveness list. A forgiveness list includes the person/people/group you are forgiving and what you are forgiving them for. The format for the items on your list is:

I forgive (name of person) for (what you are forgiving them for).

Be aware that as you write this list, you may not actually feel ready to fully forgive yourself or another; that is okay. This is an opportunity to start the process, to give energy to the idea of forgiving, and to notice who will need more attention to forgive and whom you can forgive in the moment. You will know when you have forgiven and are complete with someone or something on your list when you no longer feel a negative emotional charge when that person or entity pops into your mind. At that point you feel lightness in your being, you have more energy, and you become peace and happiness. You feel gratitude, connection, and love. Remember, you may not agree with the behavior, you are accepting of the person.

Items on your list may include the following:

- I forgive myself for yelling at my kids this morning.
- I forgive myself for complaining to my friends about my husband.
- I forgive myself for hating myself for being overweight.
- I forgive my girlfriend for always being late.
- I forgive my sister for not sending me a birthday card.
- I forgive my boss for never saying "thank you."
- I forgive my husband for having an affair.
- I forgive the politicians whose positions I disagree with.
- I forgive terrorists for not knowing that we are all connected and that our true enemies are hatred and fear.
- I forgive my father for his alcoholism.
- I forgive Mrs. Smith, my art teacher in elementary school, who told me, in front of the whole class, that my drawing was the worst in the class.

DAY 2: Write a forgiveness letter to yourself. This is a genuine, loving letter from you to you in which you forgive yourself for all of the things you have been blaming yourself about, all of the things you regret and feel guilty about, all of the self-abusive thoughts you have had about yourself that you *thought* were true. Use the items on your forgiveness list as a place to start; others may pop up once you begin writing. As you write this letter, you may reactivate some old hurt feelings. Allow yourself to feel them and continue to forgive yourself for the abusive beliefs and actions you directed toward yourself. Write whatever comes to your mind, as this letter is for your eyes only. As you are impeccable with your words and honest with what you are feeling, you will move through these old stories about yourself that blocked the flow of love in your life. When you've completed your letter, read it aloud until you feel the energy of forgiveness moving through your being, which may take more than one reading, more than one day.

DAY 3: Write a forgiveness letter to someone else on your list, and then write the response you'd like to receive from him or her. As you do this, your perception of this person will change, and you will see the circumstance that had been the cause of so much pain for you in a different light. Read your letters aloud, burn them, and use the ashes as fertilizer in a plant, knowing that you are nurturing new possibilities in your relationship with the person you are writing to. (This letter can be written to people who have passed on as well as those who are alive.)

DAY 4: Write your thoughts about forgiveness. What does it mean to you? What have you learned from focusing on it? What blocks you from forgiving? What do Jesus's words from the cross, "Forgive them, they do not know what they do," mean to you? How can you use his lesson in your life?

DAY 5: Choose someone from your list and visualize or imagine a forgiveness conversation with him or her. You may want to audiotape the following visualization and then play it as you do the exercise:

1. Sitting in a chair, make yourself comfortable, with your feet flat on the floor and your hands resting gently on your thighs.
2. Close your eyes.
3. Focus on your breath: breathe in a sense of calm and relaxation and exhale into comfort and relaxation. Repeat this five times.
4. Using the full resources of your imagination, see yourself in a special sacred space. This may be a place you have actually been or simply a creation of your imagination. Notice how your sacred space looks. Where is it? What's in it? What colors do you see? With a clear sense of your sacred space filling your being, step into your sacred place, making yourself comfortable, sitting down, and relaxing.
5. Continue to feel comfortable and relaxed. In your mind, repeat the following words: "In order to let go of blocks to the flow of love in my life, I am ready and willing to forgive. I know that through the act of forgiving, I free myself from the past and open myself to the experience of happiness and peace of mind. Forgiveness is a gift I give myself. I am now ready to forgive (notice the name or image of the person who comes into your mind, including your own, and say it).
6. Seeing this person in your mind, tell him or her what you forgive him or her for. Leave time on the tape for your inner conversation with the person. You may use the following format:

    -   "I forgive you for _____." If you experience anger, sadness, or hurt, allow yourself to feel it, express it, and continue. (If your emotional distress is too painful, you may want the support of a therapist or coach to guide you.)

- "I wish you had _____."
- "I now know that your words and actions were the best you could do at the time and I forgive you."

7. Take a deep breath, and while relaxing your focus and keeping your eyes closed, feel a sense of calm and renewal filling your being. Know that your sacred place is always available for you—a safe and loving place to forgive and open more deeply to peace and happiness.

DAY 6: Have a forgiveness conversation. Talk with someone on your list whom you have forgiven in your heart. Call him or her or talk with him or her in person. Depending on the situation the conversation may be as simple as, "I've missed you and am sorry that we had a misunderstanding." Or the conversation may focus more on the circumstance, not to rehash it and "be right," but rather to clear the air and move on.

DAY 7: Acknowledge yourself for the powerful steps you have taken to open yourself to peace and happiness in your life. Cross off those names that no longer belong on the list and commit to having the next forty days be a time of forgiving for you, setting in motion a new habit for life.

Write your reflections on forgiving.

- What I've learned about forgiving is:_____.
- In order to be forgiving as a daily practice I commit to:_____.
- The most powerful gift of forgiving is: _____.

When I have forgiven myself and remembered who I Am, I will bless everyone and everything I see.
　　　—A COURSE IN MIRACLES

Forgiveness
When you hold resentment toward another, you are bound to that person or condition by an emotional link that is stronger than steel. Forgiveness is the only way to dissolve that link and get free.
　　　—CATHERINE PONDER

week 13:
Spend Time with a Pet

There is no psychiatrist in the world like a puppy licking your face.

—BEN WILLIAMS

Spending time with a pet is a source of joy, pleasure, and amusement. As I write, my sheepdog, Rosie, is asleep within inches from my desk chair. When she wakes up, she nuzzles up to me. I pet her and chat with her, and then she usually finds another spot to take a nap unless a rawhide bone or something outside captures her attention. I am her main sheep. She keeps an eye on me and that is quiet literal, since she is blind in one eye. My cat Lucy is out and about. I've been told by neighbors that she stops by their homes and visits, as she knows her way around the neighborhood. She loves sleeping on the corner of the living room couch during the day and at the foot of my bed at night, and walking across my desk and adding a few letters to my manuscript when the keyboard is on her path. She is a great stalker. She has taught me about patience and focus. I am joyously grateful having these beings in my life. Rosie reminds me daily to greet each day with enthusiasm, eat when I'm hungry, sleep when I'm tired, always be ready for an adventure when I go outside, and that hugging is always acceptable.

Pets allow for cross-species communion, and sometimes that is the best remedy for the noise and chatter that fill our minds. Whether you are mesmerized by the activity in a fish tank, in awe of the underwater world when snorkeling, fascinated by a TV nature program, delighted when swimming with dolphins, inspired by an heroic act of a four-legged creature in a movie, surprised by the articulate words of a parrot, or soothed by the cuddly softness of your favorite stuffed animal, spending time with a pet is a prescription for peace and happiness.

HOW TO DO IT

DAY 1: Notice the fauna you share earth with. The flies, the birds, the dogs, the cats. What do you see in the course of your daily life? This may mean that you have to stop yourself from swatting some winged insects as they fly in your direction.

I used to be afraid of insects, and the thought of a cockroach gave me the creeps. In 1978, as I was preparing to move to New York City, one of my biggest concerns was that there would be roaches in my apartment, no matter how clean it was. A few months before my move, I went to a workshop that was given by Dorothy Maclean, one of the founders of the Findhorn Community. She talked about every being—plants, insects, birds, animals, trees, flowers, rocks—actually everything having consciousness, and that it was possible to communicate consciousness to consciousness. I decided I would communicate with cockroach consciousness. I was willing to make a deal. It went something like this: "I won't kill you as long as you stay out of sight when I'm around. It is okay for you to be in my apartment, I just don't want to see you. When you hear me coming, scat." It worked. In the nine years I lived there, I saw roaches about five times. When I saw them, I remembered our deal, and I didn't kill them. Instead, I reminded them of our agreement.

Today, become aware of the amazing beings that coexist with you. If there are some that are scary to you, begin to change your thinking about them and make a deal!

DAY 2: Spend time with a pet or an animal today. If you have a dog, when you walk him, actually be with him, rather than going on a walk on automatic. Act as if you are spending time with a good friend. If you don't have a pet, you might stop by a local zoo or aquarium and spend time connecting with the beings there. You might stop by your local pet shelter and see about volunteering to walk the pets that are there.

DAY 3: See a movie about pets.

DAY 4: Talk with three people about their pets. Find out:

- What is special about their pet?
- Why do they have the pet they have?
- How do their pets contribute to their peace and happiness?

DAY 5: Act as if you are different animals. Give yourself some space. Start out lying down on the floor with your eyes closed and imagine that you are a cat. Stretch those long, graceful cat stretches and be a cat. When another animal pops into your mind, be that animal. You might find it quite enjoyable to move around your living room like a penguin! Play with this, allowing your imagination to be your guide.

Do this for at least fifteen minutes and notice how you feel afterward.

DAY 6: Spend time with a pet again today. Your own or a neighbor's, or make a visit to seagulls down near the water or to the birds in the park. Allow your mind to focus on communing with this being and notice what happens when you focus your attention on being with a pet.

DAY 7: Write your reflections on being with a pet this week.

- What did you notice about yourself?
- What did you learn?
- How do you feel when you open your heart and mind to being with a pet?
- How does being with a pet contribute to your peace and happiness?

From the oyster to the eagle, from the swine to the tiger,
all animals are to be found in men and each of them
exists in some man, sometimes several at the time.
Animals are nothing but the portrayal of our virtues
and vices made manifest to our eyes, the visible
reflections of our souls. God displays them
to us to give us food for thought.
—Victor Hugo, *Les Miserables*

WEEK 14:
Express Your Love

What the world needs now is love sweet love, that's the only
thing that there's just too little of.
— BURT BACHARACH

Expressing your love is the most powerful and precious gift you have to offer. It can take many forms, as in simply saying: "I love you," or sending flowers or loving thoughts to someone. During my apprenticeship with don Miguel Ruiz, the author of *The Four Agreements*, one day he said, "There are ten million ways to say 'I love you.'" Since then I have been exploring the variety of ways I can express my love and understanding the ways in which others express theirs. What I have learned is our love is expressed when we *are* love.

Our natural state is love. Often we forget this and wait for special occasions to express our love, or for someone to act a particular way, or for the circumstances to be just perfect. When we wait to express our love, we miss out on the glorious experience of being peace and happiness that is always available to us. Truly, the easiest way to express your love is to allow love to flow through you. Here are some ways to do this:

- Think of person, a place, or an experience you love. Focus your attention on it, using the full resources of your imagination. See it, hear it, smell it, taste it, feel it. Notice what happens. How do you feel? If you allow yourself to surrender into this experience, love will be flowing through you.
- Take a few deep breaths and focus on your heart. Your heart is the place where love lives. Allow yourself to feel the love that is in your heart. Imagine your love as a glorious white light that expands with each in-breath and is given freely with each exhalation.
- Listen to a piece of music, read a poem, smell a flower, and allow the beauty that is being expressed to touch your being and help you feel the love you are.

This week, express your love, starting with your awareness of love moving through you and then in giving it away. If you notice you're holding back because you're shy or because some people, in your judgment, don't deserve your love, express it anyway. We are all expressions of God, and God is love. This week, see love in everyone and express your love fully. Remember, if some people don't seem lovable to you, they may have simply forgotten that they are love. Your expression of love may be the reminder they need.

HOW TO DO IT

resource
_____

www.CelebrateSomebody.com

DAY 1: Be love. This is a choice. Even if you are in the midst of a crisis in your life, you can choose to connect with the energy of love. Put reminders around your home and office that say, *"I Am Love."* Think of people and places you love and allow thoughts of them to fill you with love. Whether or not you believe this, act as if it is true. When you are love, everything you do is an expression of love.

DAY 2: When you are off-center, stressed, frustrated, angry, impatient, experiencing hell, ask yourself the question, "What would love do here?" Listen to the answer and act on it. The answer you receive may not be what your ego thinks is the thing to do. Do it anyway. Your ego is probably what got you into the jam you are in to begin with!

DAY 3: Consciously express your love to at least twenty people today. Be creative. You may send a card to someone, massage someone's shoulders, help someone carry packages, make a romantic dinner, listen to someone in need. Remember to include yourself in this group of twenty people.

DAY 4: Live your day as if you are an emissary of love right now. You are an angel, and the message you have been sent to give is that we are love. If you are thinking you're not an emissary of love because you don't have a boyfriend or girlfriend, because you're overweight, because you hate your job, because you are an alcoholic, because you were abused as a child . . . because, because, because . . . act as if you are.

DAY 5: Notice all the times during the day that you forget that you are love, and as soon as you notice, express your love. When you look at yourself in the mirror and you hear yourself saying, "I am ugly," change that in the moment, and express your love by having a new thought: "I am love, I am magnificent, I'm great just the way I am." If you hear yourself mumbling about your coworker, saying, "He is a jerk," have a new thought and express your love. A simple way to know if you have forgotten that you are love is when you are judging yourself or someone else, when you are abusive to yourself or someone else, when you are gossiping about yourself or someone else, or when you are critical of yourself or someone else. Then you are not expressing love.

DAY 6: Talk with three people today about being an emissary of love.

DAY 7: Write about your experience of expressing your love.

- What did you learn?
- How do you express your love?
- Write a poem or essay or draw a picture that captures being an expression of love.

week 15:
Listen to Music

Music is well said to be the speech of angels; in fact, nothing among the utterances allowed to man is felt to be so divine. It brings us near to the infinite.

—Thomas Carlyle

Listening to music is a powerful doorway to transforming your experience in the moment. Music can make our feet dance, our bodies awaken, and our hearts sing. A soothing instrumental can quiet both our inner experience and shift our viewpoint of our outer world. The words of a song can give us a new point of view that can change our experience in the moment. Music is truly a universal language that speaks directly to our spirit. Listen to it. Make it. Use it as an entryway to experiencing peace and happiness.

HOW TO DO IT

DAY 1: Create a music library for yourself with an assortment of music to calm you down, lift your spirits, and get your body moving.

DAY 2: Rather than mindlessly turning on the TV when you are home or automatically pressing the play button on your tape deck or CD player when you are in your car, make deliberate choices about the music you listen to today. When you wake up and start your day, do you want to listen to something that makes your body dance to the new day, or do you want an instrumental to slowly and lightly ease you into the day? Maybe you would simply rather hear the natural music of your surroundings: birds chirping, traffic outside your window, the flush of your toilet, the flow of water through your faucet, the squeak of your closet door. Notice the instruments and the sounds of your daily life as though you are listening to an expertly composed and arranged musical masterpiece.

DAY 3: Prepare and organize an assortment of CDs, tapes, and preset radio stations in your home, car, and your Walkman so you easily have musical choices available that support peace and happiness.

DAY 4: Go to your local library or music store and listen to/take out/buy music that is new to you, expanding your musical choices. Notice how different music influences your mood, thoughts, experience.

DAY 5: Go to a concert.

DAY 6: Sing along with the music that is playing. Your voice is an instrument, so use it. Sing in the shower, hum while in line at the supermarket, notice if there is a song in your mind and sing it. What are the words saying to you? Are they a gateway to peace and happiness or are they telling a tale of doom and gloom? I remember once hearing at a wedding the words, "Heard it through the grapevine, not much longer would you be mine." I thought that was an unusual choice for a wedding reception!

DAY 7: Invite friends to bring instruments over and make music. Use spoons, pots and pans, and bottles filled with water. Play and experiment with sound. Write your reflections about what you have discovered about music this week.

· How does music contribute to your peace and happiness?
· What is some of your favorite music?

Music washes away from the soul the dust of everyday life.
—RED AUERBACH

Experiencing music, this week, has been different than I
expected. Normally it would be about the sounds made by musicians. The music for me, this week, has been about listening to
the rhythms of life. The birds chirping, the breeze blowing, the
sound of love from being with my friends and being silent. The
sounds of the sun shining on me and the world. I continue to
deepen into my happiness.
—SHANTI

One of our newer [church] members, a man named Ken Nelson,
is dying of AIDS, disintegrating before our very eyes. He came in
a year ago with a Jewish woman who comes every week to be with
us, although she does not believe in Jesus. Shortly after the man

with AIDS started coming, his partner died of the disease. A few weeks later Ken told us that right after Brandon died, Jesus had slid into the hole in his heart that Brandon's loss had left, and had been there ever since. Ken has a totally lopsided face, ravaged and emaciated, but when he smiles, he is radiant. He looks like God's crazy nephew Phil. He says that he would gladly pay any price for what he has now, which is Jesus, and us.

There's a woman in the choir named Ranola who is large and beautiful and jovial and black and as devout as can be, who has been a little standoffish toward Ken. She has always looked at him with confusion, when she looks at him at all. Or she looks at him sideways, as if she wouldn't have to quite see him if she didn't look at him head on. She was raised in the South by Baptists who taught her that his way of life—that he—was an abomination. It is hard for her to break through this. I think she and a few other women at the church are, on a visceral level, a little afraid of catching the disease. But Kenny has come to church almost every week for the last year and won almost everyone over. He finally missed a couple of Sundays when he got too weak, and then a month ago he was back, weighing almost no pounds, his face even more lopsided, as if he'd had a stroke. Still, during the prayers of the people, he talked joyously of his life and his decline, of grace and redemption, of how safe and happy he feels these days.

So on this one particular Sunday, for the first hymn, the so-called Morning Hymn, we sang "Jacob's Ladder," which goes, "Every rung goes higher, higher," while ironically Kenny couldn't even stand up. But he sang away sitting down, with the hymnal in his lap. And then when it came time for the second hymn, the Fellowship Hymn, we were to sing "His Eye Is on the Sparrow." The pianist was playing and the whole congregation had risen—only Ken remained seated, holding the hymnal in his lap—and we began to sing. "Why should I feel discouraged? Why do shadows fall?" And Ranola watched Ken rather skeptically for a moment, and then her face began to melt and contort like his, and she went to his side and bent down to lift him up—lifted up this white rag doll, this scarecrow. She held him next to her, draped over and against her like a child while they sang. And it pierced me.

I can't imagine anything but music that could have brought about this alchemy. Maybe it's because music is about as physical as it gets: your essential rhythm is your heartbeat; your essential sound, the breath. We're walking temples of noise, and when you add tender heart to this mix, it somehow lets us meet in places we couldn't get to any other way.

—ANNE LAMOTT, FROM "MIRACLES" IN *TRAVELING MERCIES*

week 16:
Give Compliments

Compliment: an expression of esteem, respect, affection or admiration; an admiring remark, formal and respectful recognition.

—Merriam-Webster Dictionary

Giving compliments is a gift of recognition and acknowledgment. Both the giver and the receiver benefit from the energetic exchange of this gift. When people are asked what contributes to their experience of happiness, the gift of recognition and appreciation, precious expressions of love, is high on their list. The challenge is that while recognition and appreciation are greatly desired, often the receiver is uncomfortable and embarrassed about the compliment. This happens in ordinary circumstances, for instance: you have recently had a haircut and someone at work says to you, "Your hair looks great." Instead of simply saying, "Thank you," you go into a whole story about how it will really look better in a few weeks after it grows out a bit. Or a neighbor expresses his appreciation for your helpfulness and your reply is, "Oh, it was nothing." That response is a direct undermining of the power of the compliment and appreciation that was given to you. In focusing on giving compliments, we direct our attention to appreciation. When I am in the midst of focusing on appreciation, I am being peace and happiness. So this week, give compliments, and if someone says to you, "Oh, it was nothing," reply by saying, "It was something to me, and I appreciate you." And while you are focused on giving compliments, open yourself to receiving the ones that are sent in your direction.

HOW TO DO IT

DAY 1: Check out the auto-affirmer website and use it on yourself three times today. Notice how you feel and forward it to others: *www.netropolis.au.com/design/affirmations.html*.

DAY 2: When you wake up and before you go to sleep, compliment yourself. In the morning as you are looking in the mirror, spend five minutes complimenting your body for its magnificence. "I appreciate you, lungs, for working so elegantly and effortlessly; "I appreciate you, my beautiful feet, for each and every day of moving me from one place to the next; thank you, ears for the great job you do hearing; thanks, stomach, for letting me know when I am full," and so forth. At night before you go to sleep, compliment yourself: thank you, sense of humor, for reminding me to lighten up; "Thank you eyes, hands, and feet for your great teamwork today."

DAY 3: Make an appreciation journal for someone you care about. Use *www.CelebrateSomebody.com* or make one of your own. This is an opportunity to express your love and appreciation. This can also be a wonderful gift for birthdays, anniversaries, Mother's Day, Father's Day, Secretary's Day, or any day you want to express your love and appreciation for someone in your life.

DAY 4: Give compliments. Wherever you are today, give at least one compliment: in the supermarket, at the post office, at work, at home, at the bank, and so forth.

DAY 5: Write and mail three compliment letters: to a family member, a friend, and someone you don't know personally who is an important influence in your life, perhaps a particular author; a celebrity whose work has inspired you; or someone in your town whom you admire.

DAY 6: Compliment people who impact your daily life so invisibly that you may not think about them regularly: the postal worker who delivers your mail, the person who picks up your trash, the bus driver who delivers you to and from work, your boss, the person who stocks the shelves in the supermarket. Make a list of all the people who make your life easier, whom you don't often see, and compliment them. If you don't see them all today, focus on complimenting them during this month.

DAY 7: Write your reflections on giving compliments.

- What did you become aware of?
- How do you feel giving compliments? Receiving compliments?
- What will you continue to do?

After my father had seen me in five or six things, he said, "Son, your mother and I really enjoyed your recent film, and I must say that you're a lot like John Wayne." And I said, "How so?" And he said, "Well, you're exactly the same in all your roles." Now, as a modern American actor, that's not what you want to hear. But for a guy who watched John Wayne movies and grew up in Iowa, it's a sterling compliment.

—DERMOT MULRONEY

week 17:
Use the Good Dishes

If I had my life to live over . . . I would have burned the pink
candle sculpted like a rose before it melted.
—ERICA BOMBECK

Using the good dishes is a metaphor for a powerful way to live our lives more fully and happily. How many good dishes or special pieces of jewelry or clothing do you have put away for a special occasion? When you do use the good stuff, are you so anxious and worried that it might break or get stained that you really don't get pleasure and joy when you do use it? How many special things do you keep under lock and key for safety?

As I drove in my car this morning, I heard a news report on National Public Radio about a special congressional committee meeting set to begin tomorrow about September 11th. A person being interviewed spoke of how the site of the former World Trade Center Towers is sacred ground because people had died there. I had just been there two days earlier and felt the sacredness of the place. As I began my morning walk on the beach I wondered, "Does it take death to remind us of the sacredness of life? What if we lived our daily lives as sacred acts?" This is what using the good dishes is about. Celebrating. Wearing our special clothes and using the good dishes simply because they are special, and when we use them they evoke a feeling of joy and pleasure in us. So this week, use the good dishes and notice how you feel when you celebrate each moment. Being peace and happiness is the honoring of each moment.

Today, Hannah (3 years old) was wearing her Christmas dress again, because, as she had explained to me, "this is a very, very special occasion." Nurse Katie was coming for tea.

Katie was one of Hannah's favorite nurses; she worked at the hospital where Hannah had her surgeries. . . .

Now, Hannah was setting the tea party table herself. Walking slowly and carefully, she carried an eclectic assortment of china plates and cups, one at a time, from the kitchen to the coffee table in the living room. She ordered the cups and plates into a lopsided circle and set a white plastic daisy and vase from her Barbie tea set in the center. Three leftover birthday napkins, a Winnie-the-Pooh and two Little Mermaids, were joined by one that said "Happy New Year," lined up end to end "so we can see the pictures on them," Hannah explained.

As I watched Hannah arrange and rearrange the items on the table, I held myself back from making any suggestions. It wasn't easy. There was a part of me, I realized, that was overly critical of everything, that wanted to teach people, especially my children, about the "right" way to do things.

Hannah was smiling and humming, every once in a while stepping back to survey her work. She was in no hurry, and seemed completely unconcerned about the way a tea party is "supposed" to look. I watched her quietly, savoring the joy she was experiencing and the care she was giving to everything that she was doing. I longed to bring the same attention to the busyness in my everyday life, to do something simply for the joy of doing it, without worrying whether people noticed or liked it.

—FROM *HANNAH'S GIFT: LESSONS FROM A LIFE FULLY LIVED* BY MARIA HOUSDEN (BANTAM BOOKS, 2002)

HOW TO DO IT

DAY 1: Use the good dishes today. Use them for your toast in the morning and your dinner at night. Set the table as though today is a special day. And today *is* a special day because it is a day of your life. Use the crystal glasses or a special goblet that you love. Put a bouquet or a single flower on your table. Admire your good dishes and let them speak to you.

As I set the table with my good dishes, the ones my mother and father were given when they married in 1947, I am filled with loving memories of my parents and of special meals. I used to worry that something would happen to the dishes if I used them. The truth is something does happen; they evoke a sense of beauty, grace, and love that radiates from them, filling my home and me with those qualities.

DAY 2: Wear a special item of clothing today. Whether it is the special night-gown you have been saving for "just the right time" or a piece of jewelry that you thought was "too good" to wear on an ordinary day, put it on, wear it, and enjoy it.

DAY 3: Wear something that says, "Life is a celebration, a precious gift." Wear those sunglasses with the rhinestones and the gold-colored glass you bought on vacation many years ago and haven't worn since. Put on the lipstick that makes your lips sparkle, get the glitter out and sprinkle it on you. And if you don't have anything like this stored away in your home, go out and buy something. Today is your day to play. Put a carnation in your lapel. There is no need to wait. Today is your special day.

DAY 4: Use the good soap, oil, and body lotion. Do you have a special way to pamper your body that you mean to do every day, and in the busyness of your daily routine you simply forget? Unwrap that special bar of soap you have been waiting to use. Or treat yourself to a new soap in a fragrance that you've wanted. Light candles in your bathroom. Take a bubble bath or a glorious shower. Use a body lotion that lets your body know, I am grateful for this glorious body. Savor this experience with all your senses.

DAY 5: Write a poem or essay about using the good dishes.

DAY 6: Make a special meal and use the good dishes. This is a meal of only foods you love, maybe an old family favorite or that delicious bread from the bakery in town. You love the way the food looks, smells, and tastes. Simply imagining eating this food makes your mouth water. Enjoy this loving nourishment.

DAY 7: Write about your experience of using the good dishes.

- What did you learn?
- How do you feel when you celebrate each day in this way?
- How can you continue to use this idea in your daily life?

If I Had to Live My Life Over Again

If I had to live my life over again, I'd dare to make more mistakes
    next time.
I'd relax. I would limber up. I'd be sillier than I have been this
    trip.

I would take fewer things seriously. I would take more chances. I
would take more trips.

I would climb more mountains, swim more rivers.

I would eat more ice cream and less beans.

I would perhaps have more actual troubles, but I'd have fewer
imaginary ones.

You see, I'm one of those people who live seriously and sanely
hour after hour, day after day.

Oh, I've had my moments, and if I had it to do over again, I'd
have more of them.

In fact, I'd try to have nothing else, just moments, one after
another, instead of living so many years ahead of each day.

I've been one of those persons who never goes anywhere without
a thermometer, a hot water bottle, a raincoat and a parachute.

If I had it to do again, I would travel lighter than I have.

If I had to live my life over, I would start barefoot earlier in the
spring and stay that way later in the fall.

I would go to more dances.

I would ride more merry-go-rounds.

I would pick more daises.

—ATTRIBUTED TO NADINE STAIR

week 18:
Seize the Moment—Be Here Now

Realize that now, in this moment of time, you are creating.
You are creating your next moment. That is what's real.
—SARA PADDISON

Seizing the moment and being here now is the point of greatest power in our lives. The present moment is all that we ever really have. Unfortunately, we often mask the present moment in thoughts and worries of the past or future. We relive past hurts over and over again. Like the tagline on the History Channel, we bring the past to life. Or we spend time imagining the past repeating itself in our future, thereby using the law of attraction to attract to us more of the same, giving credence to history repeating itself! Indeed, we are recreating history through where we focus our attention.

I am amazed at our masterful ability to have our body in one place and our mind somewhere else. It may even be happening to you, right now, as you are reading this. Your mind is wandering, and you have to consciously choose to bring your attention back to this page. When we seize the moment, we experience the wonder and mystery that is always present in our world.

Early one April, it was unseasonably hot for three days. The temperature was in the 90s. The heat was intensified because most of the leaves on the tress were still tight in the bud. I packed up my beach chair, laptop, and sheepdog and went to the beach to write. Rather than writing, I began to focus on the heat gently caressing my skin, the sound of the surf, and children laughing at the water's edge. I watched my dog running easily and gracefully with other dogs. Everything I looked at, heard, and experienced was sparkling with life. This unexpected April heat seemed to be an alarm clock sounding that woke me up to my daily life. During the next two days I noticed flowers blooming within hours, leaves opening on the trees, birds flying and singing. I felt as though I actually lived in a Walt Disney movie. Yellow, purple, pink flowers. Leaves all shades of green. Birds with red bellies and hints of blue and yellow flying in my yard, on my lane. I thought, I really do live in a fairy tale. Since that day my awareness of my surroundings has been reawakened. My ability to direct my attention to the beauty, mystery, and power of the present moment is as simple as focusing my attention on my surroundings. I am aware that it is possible to focus on the present moment and see litter on the street, hear the noise of honking horns, see homeless people in need, and feel overwhelmed and frustrated. But does it really help anyone to wallow in those thoughts? So if you notice that your present moment is filled with thoughts of what is wrong and feelings of unhappiness, do something about it. Pick up the litter you see, imagine the sounds of the car horns as music, hear them combine with the whoosh of the breeze, the song of the birds, and the jet engine above. Give the homeless person a sandwich, a smile, some loose change, or a prayer for their well-being.

One day while I was waiting for a red light to turn green, I overheard a well-dressed, wealthy looking man having a conversation on the street corner with a poorly dressed man, who was asking for money. The man in the suit was talking with the other man about Eckhart Tolle's book, *The Power of Now*, and how it helped him change his life. I smiled, grateful for this conversation reminding me of the richness of now.

We create our experience by where we place our attention. Our future first lives in our thoughts in the present. Honor your today and nourish the seeds of a bountiful future by honoring, embracing, and rejoicing in the moment, the precious present.

HOW TO DO IT

Resources

~ *The Power of Now* by Eckhart Tolle, Novato, CA: New World Library, 1999.

~ *Be Here Now* by Ram Dass, New York: Crown, 1971.

~ *Ground Hog Day* (movie).

DAY 1: Once an hour, bring your attention to the present moment. Do it by focusing on your sensory experience. For instance, I am sitting on my desk chair, and my right ankle is resting on my left thigh. My left foot is on the base of my desk chair. I am looking at my computer screen. My fingers are gently tapping against the keys on my black computer keyboard. With each keystroke I hear a tapping sound. My back is supported by the back of my chair. I hear the hum of the swimming pool filter in the background. I have a smile on my face.

DAY 2: Every time you notice your mind wander, bring your attention back to the present moment. As you relive the argument you had with your girl-friend yesterday, bring your attention to the present moment. As you imagine the rush-hour traffic later this evening, bring your attention to the present moment. As you plot against your boss who has, once again, given you a last-minute project to complete, bring your attention to the present moment. It doesn't matter what storyline you are following in your mind, even if you are enjoying imagining a great night of romance, for the sake of this practice, strengthen your ability to focus your attention on the present moment.

DAY 3: Meditate for ten minutes in the morning and ten minutes in the evening.

- Sit comfortably.
- Close your eyes and turn your attention to your breath.
- Inhale through your nose and exhale through your mouth.
- If you notice any tension in your body, breathe a sense of relaxation into that part of your body, and as you exhale release the tension.
- When you become aware of thoughts simply turn your attention back to your breath.

DAY 4: Place signs around your home and workplace that say: N O W. Each time you see one of the signs, bring your attention to now.

DAY 5: Use your present to in-form each conversation and activity you are involved with during the day. When you get in your car to drive to the super-market, stop for a moment, take a deep breath, and for thirty seconds see yourself arriving safely at your destination. Just before you begin a performance appraisal meeting with one of your employees, stop for a moment, take a deep breath, and use the power of now to visualize for thirty seconds a successful outcome to the meeting. You may see you and your employee smiling at each other at the end of the meeting, hearing yourself say, "I am glad we had this opportunity to discuss your performance," and feeling satisfied.

DAY 6: Live each moment as if it were your last. I have heard that the Angel of Death is always on our left shoulder. How would you seize the moment if that were true?

Three months before my mother's death, she was in a hospital in intensive care. Her doctor told me that being ninety-two years old, she was quite weak and death was near. One of her nurses asked to talk with me. She asked me if I knew what was going on. We spoke for a while and she said that while my mom might not pass on today or tomorrow, from her experience, my mom was letting go. The moment became alive. During the next five days, my mom stayed in intensive care. In the presence of the Angel of Death, love was alive. My mother was so happy to have her children with her. She spoke on the phone with all her friends and family. Being with her was the most loving experience I had ever known. What I learned is that the Angel of Death is nothing to fear, because in its presence, love is alive. This doesn't mean that you have to die tomorrow to feel love in the moment. It means that if we allow each moment to die, give way to the next, and live fully in the present with the knowledge that each moment is precious and may be our last, we have direct access to love and peace and happiness.

DAY 7: Write your reflections on seizing the day—being here now.

- What did you learn about yourself and the power of the present?
- How can you use these insights for peace and happiness?

There are fine things which you mean to do some day; under what you think will be more favorable circumstances. But the only time that is surely yours is the present; hence this is the time to speak the word of appreciation and sympathy, to do the generous deed, to forgive the fault of a thoughtless friend, to sacrifice self a little more for others. Today is the day in which to express your noblest qualities of mind and heart, to do at least one worthy thing which you have long postponed, and to use your God-given abilities for the enrichment of someone less fortunate. Today you can make your life significant and worthwhile. The present is yours to do with as you will.

—GRENVILLE KLEISER

WEEK 19:
Meditate

Meditation can be considered a technique, or practice. It usu-
ally involves concentrating on an object, such as a flower, a
candle, a sound or word, or the breath. Over time, the number
of random thoughts occurring diminishes. More importantly,
your attachment to these thoughts, and your identification
with them, progressively become less.

—DINU ROMAN

Meditation is a practice to quiet your mind. It involves both focus and detachment. We live in a world of sensory overload. I am often astonished at some TV stations that consist of one or more people talking, a ticker at the bottom of the screen reporting a different story, and sometimes a picture-within-the-picture of something else. It is more than I care to be bombarded with. With all of this input coming at us, it is not surprising that we are often unaware of our thoughts. Meditation allows you to calm your mind, turn away from outside stimulation, turn within, and detach from thought. When this occurs, we experience a greater sense of relaxation, clarity, and connection with pure consciousness, Source Energy of the universe. Being peace and happiness requires the inner experience of peace and happiness to which meditation opens the door.

While there are many forms of meditation, it usually involves focusing your attention on your breath, a word, a mantra, or an object, like a candle flame or a flower. Whenever your mind wanders gently bring it back to what you were focusing on. (I also think this is good advice to improve your golf score!) This creates the two-fold practice of focusing our attention and detaching from thoughts when they capture our attention. So often in our lives, rather than witnessing our thoughts and choosing where to place our attention, we give our thoughts free rein. Since our thoughts are magnets in attracting our experiences, many of us wind up with a vehicle out of control. Meditation offers the practice of noticing our thoughts and detaching from them. When applied in our daily life, meditation gives us greater power over what our minds consume and a deeper sense of peace and happiness.

HOW TO DO IT

DAY 1: If you are new to meditation, meditate for two periods of ten minutes each. If you are familiar with meditation, meditate for two periods of twenty minutes each. Use the following instructions:

· Sit cross-legged on the floor or
· Sit comfortably on a chair.
· Keep your spine straight.
· Rest your feet flat on the floor.
· Place your forearms and hands comfortably on your thighs.
· Close your eyes.
· Focus your attention on your in-breath and out-breath.
· When your mind wanders, gently bring it back to your breath. Do this for the entire time of your meditation.

No matter what thoughts hook your attention, bring your attention back to your breath. When I first meditated, I would bring my thoughts back to my breath if I noticed that I was focused on any of the following thoughts: "This is so uncomfortable," "When is this going to be over," "I hate this," *but* if my attention was hooked by vacation plans, making love, decorating my bedroom, planting my garden, my dream house, any pleasurable thoughts, I would forget to gently bring my attention back to my breath and I would tell myself, "Well, these are good things to be thinking about." I can still remember the time it occurred to me to gently bring my attention back to my breath no matter what the content of my thoughts!

At the end of your meditation time notice how you are feeling. At the end of the day reflect on the impact the two meditation sessions had on your day.

DAY 2: Repeat Day 1 meditation, focusing on your breath for twenty minutes. Arrange to go to an introductory meditation class. Look up meditation on the internet or in your phone directory, or call a local Buddhist zendo or yoga center and get information about attending a meditation class. Remember, you don't have to sign up for a lifetime. Simply explore and experiment. Go to your local library and get a book on meditation, read it, and practice the exercises. There are many audio-cassette and CD meditation programs available. Go to the local bookstore or music store and see if there is one that captures your interest. Get it and use it!

DAY 3: Do the Day 1 meditation exercise once today, and do a twenty-minute walking meditation. As you walk slowly, focus your attention on each step. When you are moving your left foot forward, say the word *left* in your mind, and when your bring your right foot forward, say the word *right* in your mind. If you lose track and say left when your right foot is making the step, gently make the adjustment in your mind. Walk slowly and mindfully. If you are unable to walk, do the Day 1 meditation a second time.

DAY 4: Do the breathing meditation or the walking meditation once for twenty minutes. For your second twenty-minute meditation practice, use a candle flame or flower as the focus of your attention, keeping your eyes open.

DAY 5: Create a meditation space in your home. It may be a whole room that is your sanctuary or simply a chair or pillow on the floor. Be creative. You may want to have artwork, special objects, a candle, incense, photos of loved ones surrounding you, or a simple altar with objects that are sacred to you. You may want a book of inspiring quotes nearby that you can read before or after you begin your meditation practice. If you travel frequently, you may want to prepare a portable altar you can set up wherever you are that evokes a sacred meditation space for you.

DAY 6: Meditate twice today in your meditation space. Choose the meditation format of your choice for two twenty-minute periods.

DAY 7: Meditate once today. After you have meditated, write your reflections on meditation.

- What was your experience?
- How do you feel during and immediately after meditating?
- How did a daily meditation practice impact your day?
- What is your plan for incorporating a meditation practice in your daily life?

To integrate meditation in action is the whole ground and point and purpose of meditation.

—*The Tibetan Book of Living and Dying*

WEEK 20:
Go on a Media Diet

We are always doing something, talking, reading, listening to
the radio, planning what next. The mind is kept naggingly
busy on some easy, unimportant external thing all day.
　　　　　　　　　　　　　　—Brenda Ueland

A media diet means eliminating newspapers, magazines, TV, radio, movies, books, and surfing the internet from your daily schedule. Notice your reaction when you consider this idea. Are you worried that you will miss out on something important? Are you experiencing a sense of loss or deprivation? Are you wondering what this has to do with peace and happiness? This isn't a commitment to eliminate these activities for the rest of your life, although after a week of this diet you may choose to make some changes in your media consumption habits. The purpose of this diet is two-fold:

1. Our experience of peace and happiness is created by where we focus our attention. Some of the activities of the previous weeks have directed your attention to being grateful, honoring the creative power of your word, and acknowledging accomplishments. You have been instructed to "see" and experience a sense of abundance and peace in your world. This week you are asked to eliminate sources of worry, drama, and anxiety. Much of what is in the newspapers, on the radio (including the words of many songs), and TV programming reinforces anxiety about the present and future. I often hear the word *television* in my mind as, "tell-a-vision," and the vision that is being told is one that is the exact opposite of peace and happiness. So if you want a greater experience of peace and happiness in your daily life, use discretion in your choice of what you allow into your consciousness. Keep in mind this is not judging and criticizing what is in the newspapers or on TV and radio, because in the act of criticizing and judging, we remove ourselves from the experience of peace and happiness. This is about making choices about the words, images, and ideas we feed ourselves.

2. By going on this diet, we allow for more silence in our lives. Often our minds are filled with the clutter of outside stimulation. We are so used to noise that we cannot hear ourselves think. Think about it for a moment. How often do you automatically turn on a radio or music when you get into your car without consciously choosing what you want to listen to? How often do you turn on the TV when you get into your house, or even go to bed and fall asleep to the sound of a TV program, possibly even the night time news, which is often a rehash of the day's earlier news? How often do you turn on the news in the morning as an automatic habit rather than making a choice in the moment? Think of what it would be like if you gave yourself the opportunity to experience silence. It would give you a chance to hear your thoughts and to make choices about which thoughts support your peace and happiness and which thoughts feed worry, fear, and anxiety in your life. Silence also provides the space in which to dream your life. In silence we have the chance to daydream, and when we daydream our vision of peace and happiness, when we daydream our desires as fully accomplished, we are supporting the creative process of creating the experience of the life we want to live.

Enjoy dieting this week, enjoy the silence, listen to the tape of your self-talk, and choose thoughts and images that "tell-a-vision" of peace and happiness—*your* vision of peace and happiness. Notice the weight of anxiety and worry lightening.

HOW TO DO IT

First, prepare for your worries, as going cold turkey on this diet may be uncomfortable.

- If you are worried about missing your favorite TV shows, set your VCR to tape them (this may give you a chance to actually learn how to do this on your VCR, if you can locate the manual that came with it!).
- If "chilling out" in front of the TV has been a source of relaxation for you, think about what else you can do that is relaxing rather than focusing on what you are missing.
- Unplug your TV, VCR, DVD (yes, this includes watching and renting movies, too), and radio.
- If your daily newspaper is delivered, simply decide a place to put it,

somewhere out of sight. To reduce temptation, cancel delivery for this week.

DAY 1: Rather than immediately filling your new free time up with activity, experience the silence. Notice how you feel. Listen to your self-talk and have new thoughts if your self-talk is critical, judgmental, or abusive of yourself or others.

DAY 2: Make a list of activities and projects you have wanted to begin. Choose one to start today.

DAY 3: Notice when you automatically or unconsciously go off your diet and get back on it. During the week I was on this diet I was surprised to discover that when my weekly newspaper arrived I automatically opened it and started reading and skimming the local news. A friend who was visiting said to me, "I thought you were on a newspaper diet this week." I realized, in that moment, that I had gone off the diet without even noticing. This was *just* my local paper! So notice when you just start flipping through a magazine, reading the newspaper headlines when you walk past a newsstand, or are seduced by a TV in a restaurant or airport—and remind yourself of your diet and get back on it.

DAY 4: Write your thoughts about this diet in your journal

- What are you learning about yourself?
- Is it easy, or is it challenging?
- What is surprising you about being on this diet?
- Are there any adjustments you want to make as you continue this diet?

DAY 5: With the increased time you have that is not being filled with outside noise, notice and make a list of your self-talk phrases and topics that are self-abusive, critical, or judgmental of yourself and others. Next to each item write phrases you can focus on that evoke the experience of peace and happiness for you.

DAY 6: Share your media diet experience with three people.

DAY 7: Write your media diet reflections.

- What did you learn about yourself?
- How did this diet contribute to your peace and happiness?
- How do you intend to apply what you have learned this week?

week 21:
Wear Your Favorite Outfit

Some people save new clothes to wear for "a special occasion."
... What is today's date? This date is special. Go put on some-
thing "special"—something you have been saving. See how it
feels.

—EVE ELIOT

Wearing your favorite outfit is a way of honoring and celebrating yourself. You may have many favorite outfits depending on the role you are "playing" at a particular time. Can you imagine how you would feel if you were always wearing your favorite outfit? Sometimes it would be those worn, comfy sweatpants you sigh into with a sense of relaxation as you feel them embrace your body. Other times it would be your special dress-up clothes. Simply seeing them on a hanger in your closet puts a smile on your face, and when you wear them, you feel handsome and dashing, sexy and beautiful, radiant and playful. For some of us, though, we are waiting to wear our favorite outfit, just as we are waiting to use the good dishes. We are waiting for the right occasion, or until we are the right weight, or perhaps we are worried we might spill something or get a stain on our favorite cashmere sweater, so we keep in neatly folded on a shelf in our closet. It catches our attention every so often, and we even take it out and try it on, but when we think about it, we decide that today, now, is not the time to wear it. It is possible when the right day finally comes, we discover moths got to enjoy it before we did!

Being peace and happiness is about actually living your life, being fully alive, engaged in this great mystery of creation. This means each of us is an artist, and our greatest creation is the life we live. One of the most powerful ways we have to create ourselves is through the clothes we wear. So wear your favorite outfits each and every moment this week, and as you do, you may discover that when you love what you wear, not to hide behind, but rather to express who you are, you tap more fully into the creative energy of the universe, the life force, and you become your greatest work of art.

HOW TO DO IT

DAY 1: Love everything you wear today. Put on the sexy underwear you've been saving, wear the goofy-looking tie your child picked out all by himself as a Father's Day gift that makes you smile. Enjoy the soft, worn denim of your very favorite jeans. Cuddle up in your terry cloth robe when you step out of the shower. Wear the hat you love that you feel a bit shy about actually wearing. Notice how you feel as you go through your day when you love everything you are wearing.

DAY 2: Go shopping. This isn't about buying—this is about playing and experimenting. Try on those clothes you always wanted to buy but didn't think you had enough money for, or were not the right weight or shape for, or to which you didn't have anyplace to wear. As part of your shopping adventure, buy one thing that is truly an expression of the artist, the lover of life that you are.

DAY 3: Wear something you have been saving. As you take it out of your closet or drawer, know this is the special day for which you have been saving this special item. Feel the fabric, see the color, admire the style. As you put it on, allow the feeling of abundance and beauty this favorite item symbolizes to infuse your being and connect fully and deeply with the special being you are as you wear your *something special.*

DAY 4: Go through your closets and drawers and separate the things you love from the things you don't. It is time to let go of all the clothes that no longer are a clear reflection of the beautiful, handsome, loving being you are. The clothes that no longer make your heart sing may very well strike up the band when someone else puts them on. Bring them to a consignment shop, donate them to a homeless shelter, or offer them to friends. If there are some items you just love and you know you will never wear again, consider hanging them on the wall as art, or cut them up and make a quilt!

DAY 5: Now that your closets and drawers are only filled with clothing you love, create a new outfit. Combine clothes you haven't combined before. Wear that brighter color to work that you used to only wear on weekends. Take a risk and wear the shirt you love that would really brighten up your dark suit that is your on-the-job uniform. Be aware that others may comment on the creativity you are expressing, and when you get a compliment, accept it.

DAY 6: Dress up for dinner, use the good dishes, invite friends over, requesting that they wear their favorite outfits. Notice how you feel surrounded by things you love, people you love, and wearing clothes you love.

DAY 7: Write your reflections on wearing your favorite outfit.

- What did you learn about yourself?
- How do you feel when you love what you wear?
- How does wearing your favorite outfit enhance peace and happiness?

One Day, Someday, Tomorrow

I am a fifty-two-year-old woman. From the time I was a preteen growing up in Manhattan, I looked in magazines, store windows, people-watched, and fantasized, thinking that one day I will dress like that, someday I will be beautiful, tomorrow I will get the perfect wardrobe.

During the past forty-two years I have had glimpses of that experience. When I did have a dress or an outfit that got a compliment, particularly from a man, I'd go on a major eating binge, often lasting months and resulting in a twenty- to fifty-pound weight gain. So there I was in my fifties repeating the well-worn phrases: *one day I will dress like that, someday I will be beautiful, tomorrow I will get the perfect wardrobe;* yearning to be beautiful and certain that I wasn't.

During the forty-two years this was going on, I was also coming to know that we are all creators made in the image of a Loving Creator, and that our creations begin with our words and our thoughts. One day it occurred to me that if I truly wanted to be beautiful it was time to have new thoughts and faith in those new thoughts. So my journey unfolded. The wait was over. One day, the Someday, was headed for today.

How do you change a thought, how do you live into a new thought, how do you embody a new thought? The starting point is waking up to the current thoughts; then you consciously make choices about the thoughts you have and create new habits of thinking. Now let me tell you about the day I embodied my new thought.

I am an apprentice of don Miguel Ruiz, who wrote a popular and powerful bestseller that I've mentioned called *The Four Agreements*. Eighty of us meet with him every three to five weeks for the weekend. On the first weekend I noticed Tatyana. She is beautiful. She basks in her beauty. She describes herself as exotically feminine—a current day Goddess. She dresses beautifully. She and I connected. I have always had beautiful girlfriends, but I simply thought they were beautiful and I wasn't. In the arena of beauty we were unequal. Men would notice them and not me. There was no competition between us, as I was clearly out of their league. I felt badly about this, but I figured this is just the way it was. Being beautiful for me, if it was possible, would happen one day, someday, tomorrow—not today. And there were so many criteria for that one day that the list was too long for me to even know all the categories. Some of them were: when I'm the right weight, when I exercise regularly, when I have a boyfriend, when my nails are all the perfect length, when my hair looks a certain way, when the moon is in a certain position, when the rainfall is a particular number of inches, when I have a certain amount of money in my bank account, and on and on and on.

On our second weekend with Miguel, Tatyana and I had an intimate conversation and we connected again. The next weekend we were together I woke early on Sunday morning. My air mattress and sleeping bag were next to Tatyana's. As I noticed her asleep next to me I began having a conversation with her in my mind. I said, "Tatyana, you are so beautiful, you dress so beautifully, you seem comfortable being beautiful—would you go clothes shopping with me?" The next thing I knew, Tatyana was awake and said good morning to me. I told her that I had just been talking with her in my mind, and I repeated the words aloud that I had said in the silence of my mind. She smiled and said that she'd love to go shopping with me. I was moving toward Today!

The next week during a phone coaching session with Rita, who teaches with Miguel, I told Rita that I had asked Tatyana to go shopping with me for a new wardrobe. I told her the wait was over, I was ready to be beautiful, to take the beauty I felt on the inside and show it on the outside. She said, "I asked Tatyana to go shopping with me also." We checked our schedules, I called Tatyana and we made a date for our Power Journey Shopping Extravaganza. July 10, 2001 was the day. I saw Tatyana twice before that. She gave me an assignment to go through magazines and cut out what beauty looks like to me in clothes and not to limit myself by thinking that I could never wear that. As July 10th approached, some doubts echoed in my mind, and I wondered if I would find anything to buy. Would anything I loved fit me? Would I be disappointed? Would Rita be beautiful and have a successful day, and I wouldn't? When I heard those thoughts I replaced them with new thoughts: I will find beautiful clothes, Tatyana and Rita will be there to help, God is my partner in this, and I *am* beautiful.

July 10, 2001: Rita and I drive to Fashion Valley in San Diego to meet Tatyana. We decide to meet in Macy's because Rita wants to get a watch, and we think that Macy's will have a large selection at reasonable prices. I am thinking that once we meet Tatyana we'll leave Macy's and our extravaganza with proceed to smaller shops and maybe Nordstroms. While I imagined that Macy's probably has a large selection I think it is too middle-of-the-road for my transformation. Tatyana appears, looking beautiful, and after hugs and giggles we sit down for some beauty instruction. She points out colors that enhance our coloring and shows us the difference between the enhancers and the colors that drain our natural color or compete with our natural coloring. We learn fast and decide to pick out some things in Macy's to try on to get ideas for what might work. We may not even buy anything this first go-round, as we are simply getting clearer about what enhances our beauty. It is Tuesday morning, and we are the only people in the dressing room.

Tatyana and Rita both tell me that the pale-green silk beaded skirt and top look great on me and that I have to buy them. When I look in the mirror all I see is how fat I am. They tell me I don't look fat at all. I know that my eyes are simply seeing what they are used to seeing and that I need some help. I ask Tatyana to describe to me what she sees when she looks at me in this green outfit. I ask her to help me see differently. I trust that I can use her eyes to show my eyes how to see me as beautiful. She says, "If I saw you walking into a room dressed in this outfit I would think: there is a beautiful woman, comfortable in her beauty. She is graceful, creative, and confident. She is open to expressing her beauty in the way she dresses and to be her beauty." That sounds good to me. Rita and I each decide to buy some of the clothes we had tried on. I go to pay for mine and discover that if I open a charge account I can get ten percent off, and that many of the items cost less than their already marked down price. The clothes, the prices, and the saleswoman are all conspiring and assisting me to step into Today. While I am paying, Tatyana and Rita discover a sale rack on which everything is sixty-five percent off, and Rita comes toward me with an armload of new clothes to try on. I go to that rack, and along with Tatyana, find more beautiful clothes to try on. Every cell of my being is saying YES—and the clearer the yes, the more there is to take into the dressing room.

Round two in the dressing room: I put on a pair of British tan pants. I put the top over my head, a dark green rayon top that feels like cashmere and embraces my body in its sensual feel. As I arrange the turtleneck and look into the mirror, the me I had yearned for, the me I had hoped would one day, someday, tomorrow be there was looking at me. She was my reflection in the mirror. She was smiling, she was beautiful, she was me, and I *saw* her! In the sacred cathedral of Macy's, the store where I bought my Girl Scout uniform as a child, magic was happening. The wait was over. I am beautiful, and I am sharing my beauty today and today and today.

—SR

week 22:
Smell the Flowers

I was not looking now at an unusual flower arrangement. I
was seeing what Adam had seen on the morning of his cre-
ation—the miracle, moment by moment, of naked existence.
—ALDOUS HUXLEY

Smelling the flowers is an expression that reminds us to see the beauty and magnificence of life. Springtime, the time of rebirth and new life, is the perfect time to literally and figuratively smell the flowers. Crocuses are in bloom, daffodils (maybe their name is really daffy-dils) are smiling, trees are wearing their Easter outfits of new buds. So whatever circumstance you are experiencing in your life, S T O P and smell the flowers. Use all your senses, see the magic of rebirth and new life in your world, taste the deliciousness of life, touch and feel the sensations of life through your skin, and smell the glorious aromas in your world. Our senses let us know we are alive; flowers are mirrors of the cycles of life. Allow your blossoms to open; allow yourself to experience the beauty and mystery of life.

HOW TO DO IT

DAY 1: Stop and smell the flowers as you walk to work, when you pass a flower shop, or anywhere you notice flowers as you go through your day. Put a flower on your computer screen saver.

DAY 2: Buy yourself some flowers, one or a bouquet, and get to know that flower. Meditate on it, greet it, ask it questions, and listen to its answers. Keep its petals as a reminder of the natural cycles of life, the creative process of all things: germination, birth, life, death.

DAY 3: Plant some seeds, in a garden or a pot, and nourish them with your thoughts and care. As a child I watched Mom take the seeds from grapefruits, put them in a pot of soil, and place it on the windowsill. Time passed, and she had a beautiful plant. She continued to add seeds to the pot as long as there was space. Last night I added three grapefruit seeds to my three-foot-tall grapefruit plant. Thanks, Mom, for teaching me to love life and to plant seeds so they may grow.

DAY 4: Send flowers to a loved one. Send flowers to a hospital or nursing home. Give your boss/coworkers/doorman/mail carrier a flower.

DAY 5: Visit a garden. Look through gardening books at the variety of flowers in the world.

DAY 6: Identify the precious flowers in your life: family members, friends, coworkers, and members of your community, and tell them how their beauty enriches your life.

DAY 7: Draw, paint, make a collage, write a song, poem, or essay about what you learned this week while smelling the flowers. Pretend you are a flower and bloom.

Some people are always grumbling because roses have thorns. I am grateful that thorns have roses.
—ALPHONSE KARR

Be like the flower, turn your faces to the sun.
—KAHLIL GIBRAN

WEEK 23:
Be Silent

*Do not the most moving moments of our lives find us all with-
out words?*

—MARCEL MARCEAU

*We need to find God, and he cannot be found in noise and
restlessness. God is the friend of silence. See how nature—
trees, flowers, grass—grows in silence; see the stars, the moon
and the sun, how they move in silence. . . . We need silence to
be able to touch souls.*

—MOTHER TERESA

Being silent is a practice that opens us to a deep connection with ourselves and the world. Most of our daily life is filled with noise. Many
of us begin our day to the buzz of an alarm clock which is quickly
replaced by the sounds of a radio or TV, which then serve as the background
to electric razors, electric toothbrushes, running water, conversations in
raised voices over the din of the beep of a microwave, the hum of the refrigerator, the drip of the coffeemaker, the sloshing of the dishwasher, and all
of this even before we have left the house. All of this noise shuts down our sen-
sitivity to the natural sounds of the universe, the swoosh of the air through
the trees, the conversations of birds, the sound of rain against our windows,
or the purr of a cat. Most importantly, all the racket keeps the still small
voice within still and small, outside the range of the cacophony to which we
have become accustomed. Being silent opens a new world to us. If it is a
world that has been masked for too long, without noise, it will initially seem
unfamiliar. This week, dare to explore this territory. Even if you have visited it recently, approach it as a visitor and allow it to show you its treasures,
which include the nurturing embrace of peace and happiness.

HOW TO DO IT

DAY 1: Be silent for ten minutes twice today. This isn't merely not talking
and turning the radio off. Place a "Do Not Disturb" sign on your door. Turn
off the phone ringer. Close the windows and shut out the street noise. Put

your computer on sleep mode or turn it off. Sit in a comfortable chair. Close your eyes. Listen to the silence. You may notice that silence is very noisy. You may become aware of a judge inside of you commenting and criticizing this process by saying, "This is taking forever; this is a waste of time; I could be doing something else right now; I'm uncomfortable sitting here," and so forth. As you become aware of this voice, detach and let go of the thoughts as you exhale. Focus your attention on the sound of your breath as it enters your body through your nose and leaves your body through your mouth. As sounds in the room hook your attention, notice them and refocus on your breath. At the end of ten minutes, slowly open your eyes, notice how you feel, and move gently and easily into whatever you are doing next. Give some thought to what you will use to let you know when ten minutes is up. You may want to set your clock radio to a classical music station and use that as your time indicator. You may experiment with giving yourself an instruction to easily and effortlessly open your eyes in ten minutes and have faith in yourself to follow this instruction. This is a technique I use and, with practice, is extremely reliable.

DAY 2: Be silent during a meal. You may have to let your family members or roommates know you are going to do this, and you may invite them to participate. Again the judge who has been keeping up a steady monologue within you may capture your attention. Notice and breathe. You may become more aware of the taste of the food, the sound of the silverware on your plate, and the conversations around you. You may experience your whole being, or you may become impatient. Notice and be silent.

DAY 3: Be silent from the time you wake up until you leave your house. Again, you may want to inform the people you live with that you are doing this. Include in your being silent that you don't turn on the TV, read the newspaper, or listen to the radio. If others in your house have put these on, focus your attention elsewhere. Focus instead on what you are actually involved with in the moment. Hear the sound of the shower, feel the water against your body. What is the sound of your razor as you shave? Use your creativity in communicating with others.

DAY 4: Only speak today when it is absolutely necessary. What do you notice? How much of your daily talk is really necessary?

DAY 5: Sit in silence for thirty minutes.

DAY 6: Be silent for the day. Let people you will be around know you are having a day of silence from the time you wake up until the time you wake up the next morning.

DAY 7: Write your reflections on being silent this week.

- How did being silent contribute to your experience of peace and happiness?
- What did you learn?
- How can you apply this learning to your daily life?

True silence is the rest of the mind; it is to the spirit what sleep is to the body, nourishment and refreshment.

   —WILLIAM PENN

week 24:
Doing Your Best

Your best is going to change from moment to moment; it will be different when you are healthy as opposed to sick. Under any circumstance, simply do your best, and you will avoid self-judgment, self-abuse, and regret.
—DON MIGUEL RUIZ

Doing your best is about taking action, accepting, and enjoying the journey along the way. Doing your best is a cornerstone of peace and happiness. Doing your best is not about always being the first in your class, winning the prize, or getting the reward, although that is what your best might be. Doing your best is about doing *your* best. Your best may change from day to day. On a day when you wake up feeling great, your best will be different than on a day when you wake up with the flu. When you are experiencing a personal crisis, your best will be something else yet.

When you make a commitment to always do your best, you use the present moment in determining your best rather than relying on an outside standard of what someone else is doing or the way you think it should be done. When you accept you are doing your best, there is no reason to beat yourself up and judge yourself because you should have done it differently. You did your best.

All too often we judge our performance by an outside standard of success and accomplishment rather than what our personal best is at any given moment. This is learned behavior. As a child you may have come home with four A's on your report card and one B+. All you can remember of that experience is your parents asking, "Why did you only get a B+ in biology?" Since that time all you have been able to see is what you don't accomplish, what isn't good enough. That simple question on the part of your parents, who were doing the best they knew how to do at the time, installed a belief in you that whatever you do, it isn't good enough.

If you suffer or are plagued with a perfectionist gene it is possible that nothing is ever good enough for you. You may constantly see your own actions as falling short of the way they should have been done, and you may not trust anyone else to get the job done. You are so focused on what is not working that you fail to see accomplishment and success right in front of you.

Many years ago, when my youngest stepson was six years old, I saw how my perfectionism was getting in the way of both receiving help and enjoying myself. I was making dinner, and it was Gabe's turn to set the table. I had put the silverware in the middle of the table for him. While he was setting the table, I was preparing the food, and my back was to him. Within a few moments he told me he was finished and was going back to the den. I said, "Okay," and continued making dinner. A few minutes later, I went to the table and noticed that he had put the forks on the wrong side of the plates. I was annoyed and started mumbling to myself, "If I want anything done, I have to do it myself. Doesn't anybody in this house know how to do anything the right way?"

As I kept repeating these ideas, remembering loads of evidence from the past to prove I was right, I heard myself and realized how absolutely ridiculous I was being. He had done his best. The table was set. The placement of the fork on my dinner table was not going to cause demerits on my permanent record. If it was so important that the fork be on the left of the plate, I could show him next time. I began to giggle at myself, enjoying how I could so easily turn the simplest situation into a major production. This was a powerful lesson for me. I saw that often the task is done and it is done just fine, but my limited idea of what is acceptable blocks my ability to see that the best is already accomplished.

When you do your best you are forgiving and accepting, and you do the best possible each and every day, whatever that may be. If you could have done it differently at the moment you did it, then you would have! So, commit to doing your best and notice how self-abuse, judgments of self and others, guilt, and shame melt away and you experience greater peace and happiness.

HOW TO DO IT

DAY 1: Any time you notice you are judging yourself or others for what should have been done differently, say to yourself, "I did my best," or "she did her best."

DAY 2: Assess your life in terms of the following areas and reflect on whether or not you are doing your best. Are you so focused on some areas that you are neglecting others? What would be a happier balance for you? Make a list of changes you want to make and make them. Remember, this is not a task in judging yourself. Rather, it is an opportunity to see if you are doing your best to live the life you desire.

- Self-care
- Family
- Health
- Work
- Finances
- Fun and recreation
- Personal relationships
- Spirituality

DAY 3: Answer these questions:

- What blocks you from doing your best?
- How can you move through these blocks?
- What support do you need to do your best?
- How can you get or whom can you ask for this support?

At the end of the day make a list of all the ways you were your best today.

DAY 4: Do your best in honoring your body today. Brush and floss your teeth. Express your gratitude for your body in your actions: wear comfortable shoes, eat nourishing food, use a great moisturizer on your skin, get a massage, take a refreshing shower, take a luxurious bath.

DAY 5: Do your best in asking for what you need. This is an area that many people find challenging. They think that their best means doing it themselves. That is a self-defeating idea. Ask for help when you need it and accept it graciously.

DAY 6: Create a "Doing My Best Credo." What defines your best? Write it, date it, sign it, and live it. Read it daily and make a copy of it for your wallet so you see it every time you reach for your money, as a reminder that this, too, is something of value. Read it to your family and friends and ask them to gently remind you of it, if you forget. And when you do forget, simply get back on the horse.

DAY 7: Write your reflections on doing your best.

- What did you learn?
- How do you feel when you are your best?
- What do you want to remember and practice about doing your best that would be helpful in your daily life?

Creed for Optimists

Be so strong that nothing can disturb your peace of mind.

Talk health, happiness, and prosperity to every person you meet.

Make all your friends feel there is something in them.

Look at the sunny side of everything.

Think only of the best, work only for the best, and expect only the best.

Be as enthusiastic about the success of others as you are about your own.

Forget the mistakes of the past and press on to the greater achievements of the future.

Give everyone a smile.

Spend so much time improving yourself that you have no time left to criticize others.

Be too big for worry and too noble for anger.

—CHRISTIAN D. LARSEN

WEEK 25:
Faith

*I tell you the truth, if you have faith as small as a mustard
seed, you can say to this mountain, "Move from here to there"
and it will move.*

—MATTHEW 17:20

Faith in the possibility of peace and happiness gives way to the reality of peace and happiness. A simple definition of faith is believing in something one hundred percent, no conditions, no maybes, no wait and see. It is not a question of whether or not we have faith. We all have faith. The question is, what do you have faith in? Do you have faith the sun will rise each day? Do you have faith that the tension in your marriage will never be resolved? Where we put our faith is what we create. If you are uncertain of where you have directed your faith, take a look at your life and your experience. Financial woes, a great job, a relationship with the love of your life, and on-going health problems—all are indicators of what you have faith in.

There are two major categories to which we direct our faith: love or fear. If we have faith in love, in an abundant universe, in a loving God, we will view whatever experience we have through that point of view. Many years ago, shortly after I had moved into a new house in the midst of a divorce, I was looking forward to Thanksgiving in my new home with friends. It would be very different from the previous eleven years with my four stepchildren and my former husband's family. There would be five of us, and I saw this as a healthy way for me to embrace my new life. Shortly after midnight in the early morning hours of Thanksgiving Day, I got a call from my friend telling me that she, her daughter, and her husband would not make it for Thanksgiving. I was so disappointed that I felt numb. Sixty percent of my guests had just cancelled. In moments, my mind did an instant search of all the times I had been stood up, rejected, not good enough. In the midst of this self-abuse onslaught, I said out loud "Okay God, Loving Energy of the Universe, I know that you don't have misery in store for me. I am turning this one over to you, and I want the best Thanksgiving ever. I don't know how you're gonna do it, but I have faith that you will." I went to sleep. Thanksgiving turned out to be a glorious day, with phone calls from family, friends, and former in-laws. Another family who had invited me out to dinner came over, and we ate, talked, laughed, and were grateful. I put my faith in love on this Thanksgiving Day, and the thought of it still puts a smile on my face. If we put our faith in fear, focusing on the worst that can happen, and gather up evidence from the past when things didn't work out, we often get to be right. Faith delivers whatever we attach it to.

Each one of us has the power to direct our faith toward the world we want. Each day, with news reports of sexual abuse in the Catholic Church, children being kidnapped, war, acts of terrorism, and greed of corporate executives, it is easy to be seduced by fear. Yet everything in our world is created twice, first in our imagination. And when what we imagine is nourished by our faith and given attention, it becomes manifest in our three-dimensional reality. We do have the power to put our faith in the possibility of our highest dreams and trust that we can move mountains no matter what the outside circumstances are. It seems to me we have nothing to lose. We die anyway, so how about putting your faith in love and acting as if it is a loving universe? You may be surprised at the love that pops up in the midst of whatever circumstances are present, like the loving phone calls on September 11 that people in the World Trade Center and on the hijacked planes made to their loved ones. This week consciously put your faith in peace and happiness. Explore, experiment, and enjoy.

> When you come to the edge of all the light you know,
> And are about to step off into the darkness of the unknown, faith
> is knowing one of two things will happen:
> There will be something solid to stand on,
> Or you will be taught how to fly.
> —Barbara J. Winter

HOW TO DO IT

Resources

~ *Faith: Trusting Your Own Deepest Experience* by Sharon Salzberg, New York: Riverhead Books, 2002.
~ *Indiana Jones and the Last Crusade* (movie).
~ *Keeping the Faith* (movie).

DAY 1: Pretend you are a computer programmer and that today you are writing a new software program to install in you. This new, state-of-the-art, always upgradable program is called, Where I Put My Faith. Sit down and write your program of where you put your faith. Here is some of my programming:

- I have faith in a loving universe.
- I have faith that my prayers are answered.
- I have faith that I can trust the guidance of my heart.
- I have faith that all circumstances are either an expression of love or a call for love.
- I have faith in the power of love to heal and soothe.
- I have faith in Pollyanna as a powerful role model.
- I have faith that I am an energy magnet and that I attract circumstances that match my vibration.

DAY 2: Practice the **F.A.I.T.H.** Acronym:

- Feel what you are feeling.
- Acknowledge the truth of who you are: an expression of the loving energy of the universe.
- Invite your consciousness to be aware of love's presence in all situations and circumstance in your life and in you.
- Trust love's presence in your life—the still small voice—that your prayers are heard and are being answered.
- Honor every moment as a precious gift.

DAY 3: Identify something you desire. Every time it pops into your mind, see it as accomplished. You want financial abundance? See the bank balance on your next statement reading $3,000,000.00. Keep in mind that you don't have to figure out how this will happen. Allow your faith to move through the loving energy of the universe. If you get too focused on how it should happen, you limit the possibilities of the mysterious ways of the universe. Remember to acknowledge anything that comes into your life that represents abundance, even the penny you find on the street! Make sure that in your imagery of seeing your desire fulfilled you experience yourself feeling happy, satisfied, and jubilant.

DAY 4: Witness and stalk yourself today. Notice where you put your faith.

If your beliefs are not supporting what you desire, change them and add your faith to your new thoughts. I was in a horrendous traffic jam one holiday weekend. I had been sitting in the traffic for about three minutes, which felt like an eternity, since my faith became wedded to being in traffic for the next few hours. I was imagining my three-hour drive turning into a five-hour trip. I noticed what I was doing and had a new thought. I saw myself arriving at my destination, saying to my friends, "I had a great, easy ride here. The roads were clear and here I am on time." Within moments I was feeling relaxed, noticing the scenery, and the next thing I knew the traffic had cleared. I put my faith in a new thought and I changed my experience.

You may be thinking, "This is just a traffic story. What about when something serious is going on?" I have heard two separate stories from friends in which they were in the midst of being robbed and mugged. In each of these cases, somewhere in the midst of the horror, they were able to change their focus. One person starting singing a chant that calmed him. Within moments, the bandits who had broken into his car stopped the car, apologized, and said that they wouldn't hurt anyone. In the other story a woman was in a vestibule of an apartment building in New York City waiting for the buzzer to let her into the building. Someone came up behind her and grabbed her, telling her to give him her money and not to scream. She was afraid. Time slowed down and as she was reaching for her purse she started saying in her mind, "I love you, I love you, I love you." The next thing she knew he let her go and ran out of the building.

DAY 5: Write a poem or essay about faith.

DAY 6: Put your faith into the possibility of heaven on earth. See heaven on earth as you move through your day. At the end of the day, make a list of all the examples of heaven on earth you saw and experienced today. Some examples of heaven on earth for me are:

- Flowers
- A smiling child
- A loving embrace
- My dog running on the beach
- A customer service person solving my problem
- The laughter of my friend
- The taste of fresh fruit

- Cars pulling over to let an ambulance get by
- The story in the newspaper of trapped miners being rescued
- The abundance of food in the supermarket

Have faith in heaven on earth; see heaven on earth and it will expand.

DAY 7: Write your reflections of focusing on your faith this week.

- What did you learn?
- What is the faith program that is now installed in you?
- What is your maintenance plan?

Take the first step in faith. You don't have to see the whole
staircase, just take the first step.

—DR. MARTIN LUTHER KING, JR.

week 26:
Imagine

*Imagination is the voice of daring. If there is anything Godlike
about God it is that, he dared to imagine everything.*
—HENRY MILLER

Imagine you are peace and happiness. Dream your heartfelt desires. Pretend you are a being of love right now. Our imagination is our most powerful natural resource. It is the starting point of all we experience. Unfortunately, out of habit, we use our imagination to reactivate our history and repeat old patterns of fear and lack rather than dream our future anew. When you use your imagination to serve your heartfelt desires, when you dream dreams that spring forth from your heart song, when you pretend, act as if, you are love, then peace and happiness are yours for the choosing. Your life becomes your greatest and most miraculous artistic creation.

Creation begins with a spark of desire. That spark can ignite because something in our life is not satisfying. We experience lack, unhappiness, and dissatisfaction, and get an idea of our heart's desire. Or in the quiet of meditation, in the silence of a walk on the beach, bathed in the light of the full moon, embraced and consumed in the loving energy of intimacy, an idea captures our attention. With the spark of desire alive, our imagination is the resource that gives it legs and begins to root our heart song in physical reality. Using the full resources of our imagination, we create an image of our desire as fully accomplished: we see what it looks like, we hear the sounds of our dream fully accomplished, we taste the tastes, smell the fragrances, and with a clear sense of our living dream, we step into the scene created by our imagination and experience our desire as occurring at this very moment. Through the conscious use of our imagination, we activate powerful thought forms that manifest when energetically charged with our faith (believing in something one hundred percent). These thought forms are like rockets that are released into the universe. And the universe greets them with one song, one verse, a uni-verse: YES. When you do this conscious imagining for a minimum of one minute per day, you create your life anew. So, imagine, be childlike in your playful ability to pretend. This is the prep work for what you intend to come to life in your daily experience. Act as if your dreams are alive right now (since they are), and live your life with the authority of your active imagination. You are the author of your life, and your imagination, if you choose, is in the service of your dreams.

HOW TO DO IT

DAY 1: Consciously use your imagination three times today to create your experience. Since we are constantly creating our experience through our thoughts, charged with our faith, the crucial component of this exercise is to be conscious of what you imagine. For example, when you wake up in the morning and think about the healthy eating plan you began, you notice that you are feeling a bit anxious about following it. Use your imagination. For one minute, focus on a scene of this desire accomplished. Use the following format to prepare your visualization:

Desire: I easily followed my healthy eating plan today and I feel terrific.

Scene of Desire Accomplished: It is nighttime, I am in my bathroom, wearing my favorite yellow cotton T-shirt and soft, blue-and-yellow striped flannel pajama bottoms. I have just put my new green-handled toothbrush down, and I see my smiling face in the mirror. I hear the sound of running water. My mouth has the fresh clean taste of brushed teeth. I am saying to myself, "Good for me! I easily followed my eating plan today. I feel great."

Use this for any situation you are going into: easily getting a parking space, writing a report at work, having a conversation with your child, making vacation plans with your spouse. Use your imagination to *live into* your life. It is particularly powerful when you notice you are experiencing some doubt, fear, or anxiety about something. Stop, identify your desire, and write or imagine a description using as much detail as possible of your desire fully accomplished (make sure to include yourself in the scene!). For one minute, using the full resources of your imagination, live the scene of your desire accomplished. Imagine a sign, "Daydreaming Allowed Here."

DAY 2: Make a collage of your heart's desire fully accomplished. Caution: do not limit yourself by what you think is possible. Allow your imagination to supply the images of your heart song. (Last night, at a dinner party, I heard about a man who is blind and skis in the Special Olympics!) This is a collage of what your dream is, not how you are going to get there. Ask yourself the question, "What is my heart's desire?" as you choose the pictures from magazines, newspapers, greeting cards, and photos for your collage. Trust your instinct as you cut and paste. Allow your collage to illuminate and articulate your heart's desire for you. Hang the collage someplace where you can see it and silently spend five minutes per today stepping into your dream.

Supplies:

- Colored paper, poster paper, blank newsprint
- Scissors
- Glue
- Magazine, newspapers, greeting cards, calendars, photos
- Imagination

DAY 3: Create your heart's desire. Draw a heart and write a specific desire in the center. Draw lines from the center of your heart extending outside of the heart all around it. On each line, write a clear description of your desire accomplished. Beginning today, spend five minutes in the morning and evening focusing on this expression of your heart's desire accomplished. As you move around your heart in your imagination, know that your heart's desire is created.

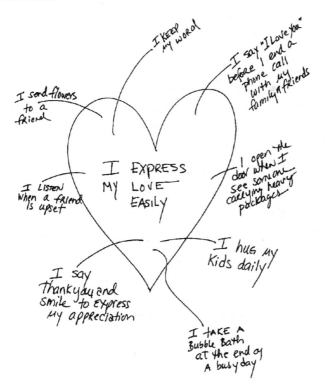

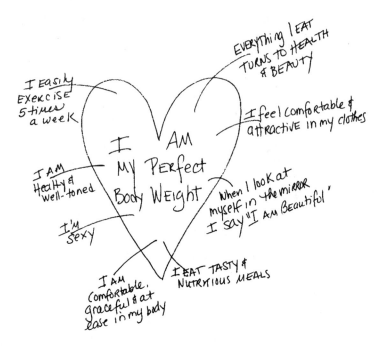

In the heart diagram:

EVERYThing I EAT TURNS TO HEALTH & BEAUTY

I EASily EXERCISE 5 times a week

I feel comfortable & attractive in my clothes

I AM MY PERfect Body WEIght

I AM HeaLTHY & well-toned

When I look at myself in the mirror I say "I AM Beautiful"

I'M sexy

I EAT TASTY & NUTRITIOUS MEALS

I AM Comfortable, graceful & at ease in my body

DAY 4: Write a letter to yourself, dated one year from today. Describe your life in the present tense, and include your dreams in this description. Read the letter aloud until you experience the joy and pleasure, the peace and happiness, of living your heart song. Burn the letter, knowing that you have participated in a powerful ritual of your intention to live your dreams. Sprinkle the ashes in the soil of a plant, and know that your dreams are seeded and fertilized.

DAY 5: Find quotes and phrases that remind you of the power of imagining, daydreaming, pretending. Display these quotes as reminders to use the power of your imagination to in-form and create your daily experience. Here are some I've found:

- Live out of your imagination, not your history. —Stephen R. Covey
- The man who has no imagination has no wings. —Muhammad Ali
- A rock pile ceases to be a rock pile the moment a single man contemplates it, bearing within him the image of a cathedral. —Antoine de Saint-Exupery
- I saw the angel in the marble and carved until I set him free. —Michaelangelo

- All men who have achieved great things have been great dreamers.
  —Orison Swett Marden

DAY 6: Listen to and read the lyrics of John Lennon's song, "Imagine," and Martin Luther King, Jr.'s, "I Have a Dream" speech. Imagine the world you desire. Rather that filling your mind with the images on TV news and in the newspapers today, imagine the world news that you would produce. See it, hear it, taste it, smell it, feel it, be it.

DAY 7: Write a poem, a song, or an essay on imagining and share it with three people. Record your reflections on imagining.

- What did you learn?
- How can you use the idea of imagining to be peace and happiness? Do it and be it.

Visualize your wishes in your mind's eye. . . . Visualize what it is you want with all your heart. See it with your inner sight and feel it as if you were really there, experiencing it with all your senses. Practice visualization every day. Our dreams help us to create our material reality as surely as our material reality helps us to create our dreams.

—Monte Farber & Amy Zerner, *Love, Light, and Laughter*

week 27:
Listen to and Follow the Still Small Voice

The Holy Spirit does not scream at us to be heard. He requires
that we be quiet to hear his "still small voice." This is such a
stretch for us, living as we do in a sound-saturated world. But
the rewards—peace, contentment, and a sense of purpose—are
well worth the effort.

—KATHY KOCH, PH.D.

Listening to and following the still small voice is a practice that leads to magic and miracles in our daily life. The still small voice is our inner wisdom, our connection with Source Energy, God's guidance illuminating our way. A challenge in listening to our still small voice is the competition that has its own ideas for the direction we take. The competition is the voice of our ego (an acronym for E.G.O. is Edging God Out) or the voice of fear (an acronym for F.E.A.R. is False Evaluation Assumed Real). A starting place for listening to and following the still small voice is our feelings. Our feelings are a magnificent guidance system that let us know if we are experiencing heaven or hell, love or fear, connection or disconnection with Source Energy, or God. If you are feeling good, peaceful, and loving, you are connected with the source. If you are feeling angry, victimized, vengeful, alone, you are disconnected from the source. When the still small voice speaks to us, in words, images, and promptings, the instruction is clear, direct, concise, unemotional, and is not necessarily what our rational mind would have us do at that moment. It may be as simple as, "make a right turn" when the quickest route would be a left turn, or "call your mother" when you just spoke with her twenty minutes earlier. The still small voice can also speak to us through a conversation we overhear that resonates deeply, or through the line in a song that gives us an idea that results in a change in our lives. This voice is always providing loving guidance; our "work" is to listen. The voices of our ego and fear are filled with emotional static and a whole saga and reasons to justify their instructions. It also is about winning and losing, having the last word, and being right.

When we listen to and follow the instructions of the still small voice, we connect more fully with universal energy. In this process prayers are answered, synchronicities and coincidences flourish. We open ourselves to the limitless source of well-being. For those of you who think that unless you do it yourself, unless you control and orchestrate all your relationships and circumstances, things won't happen, this idea of listening to and following the still small voice will seem like a big risk and will require a leap of faith. So for this week experiment, see what it's like when you ask for, listen to, and follow the still small voice. Then reflect on your experience. If you experienced a deeper sense of peace and happiness, continue with this new source of guidance in your life.

HOW TO DO IT

DAY 1: Relax and invite the still small voice to speak to you and write for fifteen minutes. Use the following instructions:

- Make yourself comfortable. Have your journal, notebook, or paper and pen nearby or sit in front of your computer.
- Close your eyes and focus on your breath. Breathe in a sense of calm and relaxation and exhale fully and completely. Do this five times.
- Feel yourself fully supported by the chair you are sitting on.
- Focus your attention on your intent: "I choose to hear my still small voice."
- Focus your attention on your heart, knowing that the still small voice speaks from your heart.
- Listen.
- When you feel ready, and trust that you will know when you are ready, begin to write for fifteen minutes. Write whatever comes to mind, even if it is, "I don't know what to write." Simply write and know that through this process, you are connecting fully and deeply with the still small voice.
- When you have written for fifteen minutes, notice how you feel.

DAY 2: Make yourself comfortable, preferably sitting up. Close your eyes and quiet your mind by focusing your attention on your breath. Think of a situation you would like guidance about and formulate a question. You can choose something you have been struggling with and are worried about, or something as simple as what to cook for dinner tonight. This is an exercise to strengthen your conscious connection with the still small voice. Here are some sample questions:

- How can I be more loving in my relationship with my husband?
- What is the best way for me to approach my boss about a raise?
- What is my heart's desire?
- How can I experience a greater sense of well-being in my life?
- What's the best birthday present for me to buy my girlfriend?
- How can I be most helpful to my brother-in-law who is struggling with alcoholism?
- What's a great dinner I can make for my family tonight?
- How can I best contribute to peace on earth?

Ask your question and then listen to the answer. If you hear something you don't understand, simply ask for clarification. Allow the still small voice to speak and listen. You may want to write what you heard to reinforce the message in your consciousness. Acknowledge yourself for asking and listening.

DAY 3: Once an hour, in the course of your daily activities, ask for guidance and listen to the response from the still small voice. Follow the guidance. Some questions you might ask are:

- What's the best use of my time right now?
- What do I want for lunch?
- What's the best route for me to take to get to work?
- Who can I ask for help regarding _____?
- Where did I put my keys?

Allow yourself to play with this. This is a communication exercise that will open you to a source of wisdom with your best interests in mind. Notice if you want to negotiate with the guidance you are getting, and then follow the guidance anyway!

DAY 4: Choose something you would like your still small voice to help you with. Ask for the help. Listen to the answer and follow the guidance. I was lazy about flossing my teeth and I thought it was important for me to floss. Not because I *should* but because I want to take care of my teeth. I noticed that when it came time to floss at night, I would begin to make deals (who was I actually making them with?). One day, I decided to enlist the help of the still small voice. I asked for a gentle reminder to floss, and I got it. I'd be standing at the bathroom sink, brushing my teeth, and I would hear, "Floss your teeth." A direct, clear instruction. I thanked the still small voice for the reminder, and I flossed. Sometimes, when the reminder comes, I don't wanna have to, and then I remind myself that each time I floss I strengthen the channel of communication with the still small voice and care for my teeth at the same time.

DAY 5: Establish a sign between your still small voice and you, between your inner wisdom and your outer life, so you will know when your still small voice is communicating with you. Quiet your mind and ask for a sign that represents your inner wisdom. Listen to the answer. In your daily life, when your sign appears, thank your inner wisdom for getting your attention and then follow the instructions.

I often thank the still small voice for speaking loudly enough for me to hear and clearly enough for me to understand.

DAY 6: Use the still small voice to articulate your heart's desire. Have your journal nearby.

- Make yourself comfortable.
- Close your eyes. Quiet your mind.
- Connect with your inner wisdom and ask, "What is my heart's song, my heart's desire, the best use of my unique talents and gifts?"
- Listen to the answer and pay attention to the images you see, the words you hear and the knowing you experience.
- When you feel complete with the answer you've received, open your eyes and write it, draw it, or make a collage of it in your journal.
- Starting today, live it.

Each step of the way, when you get stumped and wonder, "How do I do this?" simply use the still small voice for guidance. Your work is to stay focused on what you want. Use your inner guidance to instruct you on the direction and actions to take.

DAY 7: Write your reflections of your experience with listening to and following the still small voice.

Behind every blade of grass is an angel whispering, "Grow."
—THE TALMUD

WEEK 28:
Spend Time with a Child

*Children are curious and are risk takers. They have lots of
courage. They venture out into a world that is immense and
dangerous. A child initially trusts life and the processes of life.*
—JOHN BRADSHAW

*Grown men can learn from very little children for the hearts of
little children are pure. Therefore, the Great Spirit may show
to them many things which older people miss.*
—BLACK ELK

Spending time with a child is an open window to peace and happiness.
When we are in the presence of a newborn, we have a powerful
reminder of the magnificent mystery and magic of life. It is interesting to note that newborns don't *do* any of the things we as adults use to
determine our worth and value. They can't feed or dress themselves. They
don't have jobs or an investment portfolio. They don't have degrees or drive
the newest, fastest car. They don't base their life on a to-do list or doing the
laundry. And yet they remind us of what is truly the essence of life: mystery,
love, wonder, possibility. We delight in their presence. As they get older and
before their domestication has them doubt themselves, they are a joy, and
being with them is sometimes the best medicine for a weary soul. Asking
their opinions and listening to their answers brings lightness and simplic-
ity to our way of thinking and fully opens the window to peace and happiness. So this week, spend time with a child, including the child within you.

HOW TO DO IT

DAY 1: Notice your reaction to infants and young children today. When you
walk past an infant, are you drawn to make contact? When you are in line at
the supermarket or waiting for a bus, how do you react to the children you see?
Do you see the magic and wonder of these "new" people? Do you automatically feel a smile on your face in the presence of children?

In 1989 I was in the Soviet Union. I spent a few hours wandering through
Red Square and the surrounding streets. It was winter and gray, and the

facial expressions of the people I saw also looked gray and serious. After walking many blocks I was aware that no one was smiling, and then I saw the face of a child, the only smiling face around. I smiled and felt my spirits soar.

DAY 2: Make a date to do something with a child this week. Whether it is your child, your grandchildren, or your neighbor's child. Make a date and allow yourself to play, letting the child you are with be your teacher.

DAY 3: Volunteer to help children. Offer to read at your local library. Volunteer to help with children in the hospital. Offer to go on a trip with your child's class. Offer to do a project in your local preschool or elementary school.

DAY 4: Connect with the child in you. Find a photo of you as a child and allow your heart to open to that new being that you once were. Write a letter to your inner child telling him or her what you appreciate about him or her. Close your eyes and remember the feeling of wonder and excitement you felt as a child. Allow your inner child to guide your way today. Allow yourself to be present in the moment, seeing your world with childlike vision. Allow your inner child to play today. Get that manicure with the purple nail polish you have wanted and were hesitant to use because you are a grown-up (is that groan-up?). Have a peanut butter and jelly sandwich with the crust cut off. Allow your inner child to be your guide today.

DAY 5: Get recommendations from three children on their favorite books. Go to the children's section of your local library or bookstore. Read one of the recommended books and revisit a book you loved as a child. One of my favorite books is *Ferdinand the Bull*. Just thinking about Ferdinand, I smile.

DAY 6: Tell three children in your life that you love them and why they are special in your life. You can do this in person, on the phone, or by written note or email. Our words of encouragement and love are powerful gifts for the children in our life. Practice this expression of care. Through expressing your love, you open yourself to the experience of love in the moment. As responsible, loving adults, we have daily opportunities to let the children in our life know that no matter what their age, they are magnificent beings.

DAY 7: Write your reflections on spending time with children this week.

- What did you learn about yourself consciously being in the presence of children?

- What did you learn about yourself by connecting with the inner child in you?
- How can you use what you learned this week to experience greater playfulness in your life?
- What is the most important lesson you learned this week to enhance your experience of peace and happiness?

Children are messengers from a world we once deeply knew, but we have long since forgotten.

—ALICE MILLER

WEEK 29:
Pray

And all things, whatsoever ye shall ask in prayer, believing, ye shall receive.

—Matthew 21:12

I believe prayer is the sending out of vibrations from one person to another and to God. All the Universe is in vibration.
—Norman Vincent Peale

Prayer is direct communication with God, Source Energy, the Loving Energy of the universe. When wedded with faith, prayer is a gateway to peace and happiness. Every religious tradition has its own form of prayer which creates a bridge between us and the divine, so there is communion between the two. When we say a prayer of petition, asking for something for ourselves or others, we are asking God, the Source Energy of the universe of which we are a part, to focus its energy on our desire. When we have faith (believing in something one hundred percent) that our prayers are heard and will be answered, our only *work* is to allow our mind to be in a vibration of receiving (to experience the result we desire). The universe will provide direction and steps for us to take for our prayers to be answered.

Examples of this occur regularly in daily life. You're late for an appointment and unable to find a parking space, you say a little prayer to easily get a parking space and get to your appointment on time. You feel a nudge to turn down a street you have already been down three times, and there it is, *your parking space.* When you arrive for your appointment ten minutes late, you find out that the person you are meeting had to take an emergency phone call and will be with you within the next five minutes. It all worked out. Prayer focused your attention on your desire, and your faith opened the space for your desire to be manifest.

In 1982–83, a ten-month survey was conducted at San Francisco General Hospital on a group of 393 cardiac patients. One half of the group was prayed for by people who didn't know them, and they didn't know they were being prayed for. The other half of the group was not prayed for. The results showed that those who did receive prayer needed fewer antibiotics and less assistance with breathing. This study, described in the book *Healing Prayers* by Dr. Larry Dossey, supports the relationship between prayer and well-being, and an increasing number of medical schools are now teaching courses in religion and spirituality. So this week, do your own experiment. Focus on prayer, and notice the power of this tool in your life.

HOW TO DO IT

DAY 1: Start and end your day with a prayer of appreciation. You may do this in front of your altar, down on your knees at the side of your bed, or standing at the window looking outside at the glorious day that is beginning in the morning and ending in the night. Do this when you wake up, before you do anything else, and just before you get into bed to go to sleep.

In Judaism, the traditional morning practice includes the following parts (adapted from *The Busy Soul* by Rabbi Terry Bookman):

- Prayer of Gratitude: "I am grateful to you, dear God, Giver and Sustainer of life, for having granted me another day of life. Your love and faith in me encourage and inspire me."
- Daily self check-in. Think about your body's health and the way it functions well even when some parts of it are not. Offer appreciation to Source Energy for your physical health and well-being.
- Think about your mind and its ability to learn and be open to new ideas. Offer thanks to God for your mind and your ability to think and grow in wisdom and understanding.
- Think about what actions you take in loving service to others. What do you do to bring love and healing to our world? Offer gratitude to the Source of Life for your capacity to love and be loved, and to be a blessing to yourself and others through kindness and service.
- Experience your connection with all that is. Know that each thought you think, each word you say, and each action you do affects the whole of life on earth. Offer thanks to God for your awareness and oneness with all that is.
- Meditation: read inspiring words and reflect on how they apply to you today.
- Your nighttime prayer may be a simple expression of gratitude for all that you have been offered and received during the day. The prayer I often say as I am drifting off to sleep is, "Thank you, God, for another day of loving."

DAY 2: Use prayer spontaneously throughout the day when you notice you are off-center and feeling victim to the circumstances and conditions of your life. As soon as you notice you are aggravated, annoyed, frustrated, critical, or judgmental, say a prayer. Your prayer may be as simple as, "Loving Energy of the Universe, guide me through this challenge," or it may be the repetition of a familiar prayer, such as the Serenity Prayer by Reinhold Niebuhr:

> God grant me the serenity to accept the things I cannot change.
> The courage to change the things I can.
> And the wisdom to know the difference.

Or make up your own spontaneous prayer in the moment for the circumstances you are presented with. I noticed a few years ago, when I was driving in my car and lost, that I yelled aloud to God, bellowing "God dammit" as though I was blaming God in the midst of my dilemma. After a few minutes I realized God was exactly who I needed to call upon since my self-talk was critical of my being lost and not knowing the way. It occurred to me that I yelled out to God in a loud voice so I could be reminded to use Source Energy above the chatter that was filling my mind. I took a deep breath, laughing at myself, and said, "God, guide me." Within moments I saw a sign for the road I was looking for!

DAY 3: Take a prayer you are familiar with, one you may have learned as a child by rote, and say it, read it, allow the words to come alive in you. In the Christian tradition this is an example of the practice of *Lectio Divina*, which means "divine reading." This practice is a means of developing a deeply personal and intimate relationship with God. In the words of Marina Wiederkehr from The *Song of the Seed*:

> Lectio is a way of reading with the heart. It is a contemplative way
> of reflecting on the Scriptures or other spiritual classics. . . .
> When you romance the Word, you . . . ponder it, pray it, sing it,
> study it, love it. . . . Listen to it with the ear of your heart. Cling to
> it as a beloved. Cherish it. Become a home for it.

DAY 4: Say a prayer before each meal. This is an act of gratitude, an opportunity to connect with all that has been involved in bringing the food to us, and a chance to recognize the food for the nourishment it represents for us.

I used to feel on the spot when someone asked me to say grace. Then one day, as I sat at the table, by myself, I decided to say a prayer before I ate. I sat in silence, and this is the prayer that presented itself to me:

> I thank all the elements for bringing this to food to me.
> The Earth for the soil that feeds the plants and gives them a place
> to grow.
> The Water that nourishes the plants and animals.
> The Sun that shines its light on all that grows.
> The Air that spreads the seeds and through its breath gives this
> food strength.
> I thank all the people involved in bringing this food to me today,
> including the checkout people at the supermarket, the par-
> ents of the people who planted the seeds, the owner of the
> company who delivered the food to my local market.
> May this food nourish and expand my experience of Love in all
> that I think, say, see, hear, touch, smell, taste, feel, and do.
> And so it is.

DAY 5: Say the "Prayer for Peace and Happiness" once an hour today (see page 3).

DAY 6: Create a prayer ritual that you can incorporate into your life as a daily spiritual practice. Examples of this may include the following:

- A specific prayer you say each morning and evening
- A daily practice of appreciation for the gifts in your life
- The use of a specific prayer (Prayer for Peace and Happiness; Serenity Prayer; The Lord's Prayer; and so forth) whenever you notice you are out of connection with Source Energy
- Time in nature when you feel your connection with the natural world.
- A specific prayer time each day when you pray for the highest good for those you love and for peace and happiness for all beings

DAY 7: Write your reflections on prayer.

- What did you notice this week about the power of prayer in your life?
- How did you use prayer as a tool this week to strengthen your connection with God, the Loving Energy of the Universe?

· How do you plan to incorporate prayer in your daily life?

God scattered holy sparks all over the world. Whenever a person prays with intent, his words attract one of these sparks and propel it heavenward to add brilliance and sparkle to God's glorious crown.

—Arvei Nachal, *Commentary on the Talmud*

week 30:
Be a Visitor in Your Town

Exploration is really the essence of the human spirit.
—Frank Borman

Being a visitor in your town is a wonderful way to reacquaint yourself with the place you live. It gives you the opportunity to see with fresh eyes those places that have disappeared into the background. Being a visitor also enhances our experience of the present moment by having us pay attention to where we are when we are there. So often in our human experience, our mind is one place, our body another place, our spirit is off on its own, and our consciousness is focused in the past or future. Being peace and happiness requires our being aligned in body/mind/spirit and appreciating the moment. So this week, be a visitor in your town, "see" where you live and appreciate it—its beauty, diversity, colors, fragrances, sounds, familiarity, and discover it anew.

HOW TO DO IT

DAY 1: Take a new route and notice what you see. If you always go to the right when you come out of your driveway or apartment building, go to the left today. Take the stairs rather than the elevator. Take a bus rather than the subway. Walk rather than drive. As you take this new route, notice what you see. Actually be where you are when you are there. Stop and smell the flowers in the flowerbox of the store you walk by. Notice the stores in your neighborhood. *See* the neighborhood you call home.

DAY 2: Look in your local newspaper at the listing of community and cultural events for the week and make plans to do something new, or something you haven't done for a while. Go to an opening at an art gallery. Go to the opera. Attend a community planning meeting. Take a cooking class. Be a member of your community, and while you are participating in this activity, talk with two people you haven't spoken with before. Remember, act as if you are a visitor in your town and be open to new experiences.

DAY 3: Get to know your neighborhood merchants. Go into a store you usually shop in and a store you haven't been in before and chat with the people working there. You might do this at your supermarket. Go to a checkout line with a cashier you don't know and have a conversation. Focus your conversation on something you appreciate or a question you have *as a visitor.* Remember, the purpose of this is to experience peace and happiness, so don't complain about long lines or lousy weather!

DAY 4: Today be a visitor in your house or apartment. If you always sit at a particular seat at the dining room table, switch. If you usually sit in a particular chair, move the chair to another place in the room or sit somewhere else. Tonight, sleep on a different side of your bed. Again, be awake and aware of your surroundings. See your home through eyes of appreciation. Be peace and happiness in your home. If you notice that you are dissatisfied with where you live and mainly focus on what you don't like, make some changes. Buy a bouquet of flowers or a new plant. Change the furniture around. Be a visitor in your home as if this is a desired place you planned to visit.

DAY 5: Get a local map and plan an exploration of your town. Go to a park you have never gone to before. Drive through an unfamiliar part of town. Plan excursions down new streets to places you've never been before.

DAY 6: Today expand your experience of being a visitor and play with the idea of being a visitor to planet earth. What are the customs you notice? What are the costumes people wear? What do they eat? What language do they speak? What do you notice when you are a visitor on planet earth?

DAY 7: Write a letter and send it to your local paper or chamber of commerce expressing your appreciation for your town. Write your reflections of your experience of being a visitor in your town.

- How did acting as if you were a visitor change your perspective of where you live?
- What did you learn about your town?
- How do you feel about your town after being a visitor for a week?
- How can you continue to experience your town and your home as great places to be?

A Visit to New York

I was born and raised in New York City. I live on Long Island now and work in the city one or two days per week. I am comfortable in Manhattan and know my way around. Often because of this familiarity I don't visit the city. I go there, do what I have to do, see friends, and go home. Last week I was a visitor. I sat on the bus looking out the windows, noticing the magnificent greens of the new leaves on the trees. I stood in Times Square in awe of the neon signs. Particularly the one, high above all the others, that read: "Imagine all the people living life in peace." Slowly, I turned looking in one direction after the other. The beauty of this creation inspired me. The sound of the steel drums, the amazing break-dancing, the musicians from Bolivia were spectacular street theater. Being a visitor, that simple shift in perspective, is the best way to be wherever I am. Being open to new sights actually evokes new sights, new experiences, truly a greater experience of peace and happiness.

—SR

week 31:
Exercise

Exercise: the act of bringing into play or realizing in action; a regular or repeated use of a faculty or bodily organ; a drill carried out for training or discipline.

—*Merriam-Webster Dictionary*

Exercise is a way to train our body and our mind. Often times when we hear the word *exercise* we automatically think of physical exercise. The word is also applicable to the training and discipline of our mind. Professional athletes repeatedly tell stories of the importance of training both their minds and bodies (for example, Olympic skiers who practice their ski runs in their minds as preparation for actually skiing the slope). When you participate in physical activity for fitness purposes, exercising your mind, seeing yourself as accomplishing the desired result, seeing the muscle you are exercising, is the foundation for excelling in your body. Exercise is a repeated action or discipline that strengthens a muscle, whether the muscles are your abdominals, your lower back, or your muscle of appreciation, expressing your love or peace and happiness.

What is crucial in strengthening your muscle is a regular practice, otherwise known as an exercise program. Often the greatest challenge to a regular practice is creating a new habit pattern. Human beings follow the path of least resistance. This means that we follow the path of well-trod habits in our thoughts, words, and actions. When we choose to make a change in our lives, whether it's a regular physical exercise program, saying a prayer before each meal as an expression of appreciation, or listening to and following the still small voice within, we have to be disciplined to create a new habit pattern. When the pull of the old habit gently calls to you and starts negotiating (come on, it's okay not to go to the gym today, go tomorrow, stay in bed where you are so comfortable, and so forth), exercise your discipline and do the new behavior.

HOW TO DO IT

resource

~ *8 Minutes in the Morning* by Jorge Cruise, New York: Harper Collins, 2001.

DAY 1: Plan a physical exercise regime for this week. If you already do physical exercise regularly, when you do it this week pay particular attention to being present and awake. When you are strengthening your triceps, feel your triceps. Pay attention to your breath, using your exhalation to let out tension as you exert yourself and allowing yourself to renew and refresh with each inhalation. When I first began weight training, I looked forward to the time of rest between the ten or twelve repetitions of each exercise I did. After many months of this focus, it occurred to me I could rest on each inhalation, so I got to rest more frequently than I had when I was waiting to complete the reps. If you have not been exercising regularly, plan to do so this week. Even if you simply walk around the block three times this week, create a physical exercise plan and notice what you think and how you feel when you are doing it.

DAY 2: Create a mind exercise program to practice this week. The purpose of this is for you to be more aware of what your thoughts are and to be thinking thoughts that are supportive of yourself and others. If you are someone who often complains about other drivers, or the weather, or not having enough time, then this week exercise new thoughts about these topics.

DAY 3: Stretch your body. Stretching increases our flexibility. If you are not sure of the appropriate form, go to a stretch class at your local gym or rent an exercise video with a stretching section. Be gentle with yourself, use your breath to deepen your stretch, and focus on the stretch you are doing as you do it. If you notice your mind wandering, bring your attention back to your breath and your body. If you notice you are holding your breath, release it and gently relax into the stretch. Let your body be your guide.

DAY 4: Stretch your thoughts. Practice the idea that everything you do and that others do is the best they can do at the moment. If they could have done something else, they would have. When I practice this exercise, I strengthen my muscle of acceptance of myself and others, and I am more deeply connected with peace and happiness.

DAY 5: Create a physical exercise plan to practice for a month. You may sign up for a class, join a gym, use your treadmill that has gotten dusty, or make plans with a friend to jog after work. In your calendar or your Palm Pilot, schedule the days you will exercise. During this month, do it. Part of my exercise program is walking a mile and a half on the beach with my dog. Some days I get to the beach, and I don't wanna do the walk. I hear a whiny voice inside me giving reasons why I don't have to walk a mile and a half, but when I start putting one foot in front of the other, I begin to notice the sun glistening on the water and feel the sand beneath my feet. In a very short time, I notice I am half-way done, and I feel energized and happy. I've learned that doing the exercise when I initially don't want to strengthens the physical exercise habit in my life. If there is a day when I am not feeling well, I honor that. I use my body as my guide rather than listen to the whiny voice of sloth and laziness!

DAY 6: Exercise your mind today by spending two ten-minute periods of time in silence.

- Sit comfortably.
- Close your eyes.
- Focus on your breath, inhaling and exhaling.
- When your mind wanders focus on your breath allowing yourself to quiet your body and mind.

DAY 7: Write your reflections on exercising this week.

- What did you learn about yourself?
- How can you incorporate exercise for your body and mind in your daily life?

week 32:
Use Your Feelings as Your Guide

Feelings are your personal guidance system.
—SR

Using your feelings as your guide is the most direct indicator of whether or not you are being peace and happiness. Our feelings are a foolproof guidance system, letting us know if we are experiencing heaven or hell, love or fear, well-being or dis-ease. This does not mean we are good people if we have "positive" feelings and bad people if we have "negative" feelings. The truth of who we are is always that we are expressions of God, Source Energy made manifest. We are made in the image of the creator and just because we forget that, it doesn't mean it is not true! Quantum physics has now demonstrated what ancient wisdom has taught through all time, we are energy. Another way of expressing this idea is that we are spiritual beings having a human experience.

Think of your body as an instrument, and just as musical instruments come in all sizes, shapes, and colors, so does our human instrument. All instruments have a wide range of sounds, some on-key and some off. It is the same with people. When our instrument is being played with the greatest ease and flow, we are vibrating at a frequency of well-being, and our sound is a joy to hear. Our feelings let us know when we are in tune or out of tune. When a musical instrument is out of tune, it is adjusted, and while some time might be spent on the "story" of why the instrument is out of tune, the major focus is on the sound and returning to being a finely tuned instrument. It seems as if human beings spend much more time on the "story" of why their instrument is out of tune than simply doing a "tune-up."

Have you noticed that when someone asks you how you're feeling, or you ask others how they are feeling, a usual response is a detailed explanation of what is going on in their lives, often a retelling of stories long over, dramas, some tales of woe that may actually have been resolved? Since our experience is shaped through the law of attraction, the more we repeat, retell, reactivate stories of woe, the more we use them as the seeds of our future and the fruits of our present. Another common response is when people say they are fine, when their inner experience is one of anxiety and dismay. In

terms of the law of attraction, we attract according to our energetic vibration, and if there is a discrepancy between our words and our vibration,
vibration wins and is the attracting magnet.

You may be thinking, "Sure, sure, sure this is easy to talk about but my
feelings are real." Precisely—your feelings are real. It is the meaning that you
give to them, the stories that you tell and believe that is putting the cart before
the horse. The cart is the story, and since we are meaning-making machines,
we make up our stories based on the patterns of thought and stories we have
learned from our parents, teachers, and the collective consciousness of the
planet. We can make up new stories in each and every moment. Our feelings,
which never lie, tell us in the moment how we are vibrating. When you are
suffering, in hell, feeling anxious, frustrated, angry, impatient, hopeless, or
helpless, your feelings, the sensations you feel in your body, are simply letting you know you are out of tune. Not whether you are good or bad or worthy
or unworthy—these are human interpretations, stories you are making up!
It is, therefore, very important to feel your feelings, whatever they are, and
once you feel them, I repeat O N C E you feel them, use them as a spring-
board to tune your instrument. There is no need to judge yourself if you have
what is called a "negative" feeling. It is simply a reminder that you are out of
tune. Positive feelings are indicators that you are finely tuned. Simply put, we
are either in flow with Source Energy (instruments of love) or out of connection with Source Energy (off-key, off-center, out of tune). Which would
you rather be? Use your feelings as your guide and peace and happiness as
the point of view in the stories you create, and notice your heart song vibrating through you. Not only does this enhance a personal experience of well-
being, it has a direct impact on our contribution to the collective consciousness
of the world. So let your feelings be your guide.

HOW TO DO IT

DAY 1: Notice what you are feeling. Check in with yourself once an hour.
What are you experiencing? What sensations are you feeling in your body?
Remember this is *not* what you are telling yourself about what you are feeling, simply what you are feeling. "I feel comfortable in my body, my breathing is full and deep, I have a smile on my face, I feel a tightness in my chest,
there is a dull pain in my the lower right side of my back."

Today is your day to become aware of how your body feels. Any time
you notice tension in your body, breathe into that part of your body and

allow the tension to be released into the earth as you exhale.

DAY 2: Notice what you are feeling regarding your emotions. Check in with yourself once an hour. Are you calm, content, joyful, overwhelmed, anxious, angry, or scared? Notice what you feel and simply feel the feeling.

DAY 3: Allow your feelings to be your guide, and when you are off-center, out of tune, experiencing hell, use the following technique:

· Acknowledge what you are feeling in the moment (I am feeling frustrated and overwhelmed, with sweaty palms and tension in my stomach).
· Choose what you would prefer to be feeling (I choose to feel calm and focused, comfortable in my body).
· For thirty seconds, imagine something that evokes the feeling you want to feel ("It's 3:00 P.M. I am lounging on a comfortable beach chair on the beach in East Hampton. I am watching the gentle flow of the waves, feeling the sun-drenched breeze on my body.") It is usually easier to imagine a scene unrelated to the content of what is causing your agitation. The purpose of this exercise is to develop your ability to change your vibration at the point of your greatest power—N O W.
· Continue on with your life (cooking dinner, paying your bills, taking a bath, driving to work, and so forth).

DAY 4: Allow your feelings to be your guide, and when you are off-center, out of tune, experiencing hell, use the following technique:

· Acknowledge what you are feeling in the moment (angry, tension in my temples, a frown on my face, my heart is pounding in my chest).
· Choose what you would prefer to be feeling (calm, my heart beating gently, a smile on my face, at ease, confident).
· Ask yourself what you believe about the current situation that is creating the feeling you are having ("I am afraid I'm not going to get to my job interview on time, and I will screw up getting this new job before I even get there," or "I believe I am helpless in dealing with my health problems," or "I believe I am never going to be in a satisfying relationship," and so forth).
· Make up a belief that supports the way you want to feel and focus your attention on your new belief ("I have a great job interview, I deserve

having the job of my dreams. I have support and excellent care in experiencing well-being in my life. I am in a loving marriage.")
· Continue with your day.

DAY 5: During the day, whenever you notice you are feeling like a victim or that you are a victimizer, make up a new story about the circumstances you are in. For example, try a story in which you are a finely tuned instrument and everything is perfect the way it is. I was recently feeling like a victim and plotting revenge about something going on in my home. I noticed I had a desire to tell others the drama. So I vented to a friend, who did not get seduced by the story, and once I did that, I remembered that continued focus on the story was simply that, continued focus on the story. I asked myself, "What would love do here?" I kept being pulled back in my mind to the drama, and I kept asking, "What would Love do here?" Within moments I felt calmer and thought, "We all did the best we could do."

Later on, as I was sitting quietly, I had memories of similar circumstances in my life, and I was tempted to use them to get back into the drama. Instead I asked, "What would love do here?" And I followed the advice I heard from my still small voice. I was loving, in the tone of my voice and in my thoughts. Within a few hours I had moved through this experience and had also let go of past baggage. I let my feelings be my guide, and when my feelings indicated I was off-key, I did a tune-up. I needed many tune-ups during those hours, so I got them! During the next two days, I was repeatedly tempted to tell the story about what had happened and what I had learned. I knew the temptation was more about habit than anything else and there was no need to tell the story, only to express my love.

DAY 6: Create your own set of procedures to use when you need a tune-up. What are operating instructions you can follow? Put these instructions in a place where you can see them and then use them. Every time you use them, give yourself a pat on the back. Know you are creating a new pattern, one that includes regular check-ups and maintenance to keep your instrument finely tuned. Update your operating instructions as necessary.

DAY 7: Write your reflections of using your feelings as your guide.

· What did you learn?
· How can you use what you learned so that peace and happiness is the dominant tune you sing?

week 33:
Take a New Path

Whenever I draw a circle, I immediately want to step out of it.
—R. Buckminster Fuller

Taking a new path awakens us more fully to the present moment. Human beings follow the path of least resistance. This idea in action is seen in the habit patterns we follow in the course of our daily life. For example, your alarm clock goes off, as you reach for the snooze button, with your eyes closed, you think, "just five more minutes," and roll over. The next thing you know your alarm clock is beeping again. You get out of bed, your eyes are partially open as you go into the bathroom, pee, brush your teeth, turn on the shower, step into the shower and sigh as you feel the water against your body. This is a routine, a well-trod path. Habit patterns provide a structure that enables us to easily perform routine things. The danger is we often continue with the habit pattern because we are used to it, even when it is no longer effective and satisfying.

In addition to habits in our actions, we have habit patterns of thoughts and words. We think and say them on automatic. The idea of taking a new path is to be awake to our patterns and create new pathways in our thoughts, words, and actions when the old ones no longer contribute to peace and happiness.

HOW TO DO IT

DAY 1: Take a new path to the places you go. Drive down a different road on your way to work. Take a bus instead of the car; park your car a few blocks from where you are going, and walk the rest of the way. Use the stairs at work instead of the elevator. Pick the kids up from school today rather than having them take the school bus. Play with this. Be creative.

DAY 2: Change the way you normally do things. If you always brush your teeth before you shower, today take your toothbrush into the shower with you and brush your teeth in the shower. If you usually automatically turn on the radio when you are fixing breakfast, today leave the radio off, and listen to the sounds of your home in the morning. Are birds singing, are your kids laughing, is there an argument you can hear, what does the sound of running water sound like? Sit at a different place at your table. Experiment writing with your nondominant hand. Sleep on the other side of the bed. Put your watch on the other wrist. Play with taking a new path.

DAY 3: Do something different with what you wear. Wear the sexy underwear you've been saving. Shave, or don't shave. Wear your hair down, if you usually wear it up. Wear a tie that makes you smile rather than the one you always wear with your corporate uniform. Paint your fingernails with the gold glitter nail polish that makes you smile when you see it on your daughter's fingernails. Wear no make-up for the day. Play. Enjoy. Take a new path.

DAY 4: Follow the path of your thoughts and think happy thoughts today. When you notice that your thought patterns are taking you down a road that is hellish, have a new thought. Notice, when you put your mind to it, that you can turn lemon thoughts into refreshing lemonade.

Recently, as I was leaving a friend's house after having visited over a holiday weekend, he said to me, "Get ready for a long drive; you're going to get into a lot of holiday traffic." That's not the farewell idea that I wanted to be thinking as I began my journey home. I went over to him and said, "Imagine that I have an easy, smooth drive home and that I call and let you know that traffic was light and my drive was relaxing." Having a new thought, creating a new pathway in our thinking is magical. Experiment. (And I did have an easy drive home. I even got on an earlier ferry!)

DAY 5: Create a new path in your life that opens the door wide to peace and happiness. Here are some examples:

- Signing up for a regular yoga class
- Beginning each day with an inspirational reading
- Enjoying the quiet of each morning by not automatically turning on the morning news
- Taking a bubble bath before you go to sleep
- Scheduling a regular massage
- Writing an appreciation list of what you are grateful for before you go to sleep
- Buying a subscription to your local theater program.

Let your heart be your guide as you create this new path in your life.

DAY 6: Do something you have been putting off or have been *afraid* to do. Get your hair colored. Buy and wear those rose-colored sunglasses. Have a makeover at the make-up counter in your local department store. Get home before your wife, fill your bedroom with candles, and have a romantic dinner in bed. Audition for the play in your community theater. Join the choir. Wear a sexy outfit. Express your ideas at work. Talk to that person in the gym you think is so attractive.

DAY 7: Write your reflections about taking a new path.

- What did you discover?
- How can you use this idea in your daily life?
- How does taking a new path illuminate peace and happiness?

Autobiography in Five Short Chapters

CHAPTER ONE

I walk down the street.
　　There is a deep hole in the sidewalk.
　　I fall in.
　　I am lost. . . . I am helpless.
　　　　It isn't my fault.
It takes forever to find my way out.

CHAPTER TWO

I walk down the same street.
　　There is a deep hole in the sidewalk.
　　I pretend I don't see it.
　　I fall in again.
I can't believe I am in this same place.
　　　　But it isn't my fault.
It still takes a long time to get out.

CHAPTER THREE

I walk down the same street.
　　There is a deep hole in the sidewalk.
　　I *see* it is there.
　　I still fall in . . . it's a habit . . . but,

my eyes are open.
I know where I am.
It is *my* fault.
I get out immediately.

CHAPTER FOUR

I walk down the same street.
There is a deep hole in the sidewalk.
I walk around it.

CHAPTER FIVE

I walk down another street.

—PORTIA NELSON

week 34:
Ask for Help

We cannot climb up a rope that is attached only to our own belt.

—WILLIAM EARNEST HOCKING

Asking for help and receiving support are necessary habits for peace and happiness. Most people have difficulty establishing this habit pattern. We often like to help others and don't like to ask for help from others. We seem to be attached to an idea that we will have a higher score on our permanent record (where is this permanent record, anyway?) if we do it ourselves. We don't want to bother others or be indebted to them. We focus our attention on how our request for help will be a burden to the person we are thinking of asking, so we don't ask for help, and we wonder why people don't help us the way we help them. Then we get angry at ourselves or at the person we never asked for help! The flow of love requires both giving and receiving, asking and allowing. Help, resources, abundance, and miracles are available to us simply by asking, wrapped in faith (believing in something one hundred percent) and allowing ourselves to receive. This is true in all areas of our lives, whether it is asking for help carrying heavy packages, stopping at a gas station to ask for directions, asking a friend for a shoulder to cry on, asking a credit card company for a new payment plan, and asking God to guide you through a dark night of the soul. The more you ask, the more you receive, the more connected you feel, and the more you have to offer.

HOW TO DO IT

DAY 1: Make a list of the kinds of help you'd like to receive, for example, help with carrying packages, keeping the house in order, a shoulder to cry on, or help with a new perspective in seeing a situation or circumstance. Be creative. Identify whom you might ask for each type of help.

DAY 2: Just do it. When you need help, ask for it. If the person you ask is unable to help you, remember it doesn't mean you shouldn't have asked and that no one wants to help you. It simply means that person wasn't available to help you. So ask someone else.

DAY 3: Acknowledge yourself when you ask for help, "Good for me! I asked for help." This will create a new pattern, making it easier for you to ask for help again in the future.

DAY 4: When you ask for help and it is given to you, receive it. Simply say, "Thank you." You do not owe the person who helped you. In a true helping relationship, both the receiver and the giver benefit.

DAY 5: Help someone and notice how good you feel for having been helpful. Remember, when you ask others to help you, you give them the opportunity to have that good feeling.

DAY 6: Continue asking for and receiving help.

DAY 7: Write an essay, poem, or words of wisdom about your experience asking for help.

- What did you learn about asking for help?
- What blocked the flow of asking?
- What made it easier for you to ask for help?
- What is the most important lesson you learned about asking for and receiving help?

week 35:
Take a Vacation

*Vacation: a period of time devoted to pleasure, rest or relax-
ation; freedom from occupation; to be empty, at leisure.*
—AMERICAN HERITAGE DICTIONARY OF THE
ENGLISH LANGUAGE

Taking a vacation, whether for an hour on a massage table, a long weekend at the beach, or a three-week holiday exploring foreign lands, is an entry point to peace and happiness. I took a vacation this morning. I hadn't realized as I drove to meet a friend that our morning walk in the woods with our dogs would be a vacation, but it was. We parked our cars, set off on the trail, not sure of where the path would lead us. It was one of those glorious summer mornings, sunny, clear, a breeze in the air. Ah, the joy of a new day, the beauty of nature.

As the trail became sandy, we thought we would soon be approaching the bay. And there it was. We weren't quite sure where we were, so we explored. And then she said, "You wanna go into the water?" My immediate reaction was, it's too chilly, we don't have towels, and then a surge of adventure filled me, and I said, "Yes." There we were in the water, wearing an assortment of underwear and workout clothes, and she called out, "I'm on vacation." A few miles from our homes, we were on vacation, experiencing pleasure and relaxation. So often the demands of daily life leave us depleted. Yearning for the weekend to catch up on some rest, dreaming of the vacation we'll take next week, next month, or next year. Then we are so wound up that by the time we get into the rhythm of our vacation, it is time to go home again.

It seems to me that vacations start with our state of mind rather than a location change, although a magnificent location can certainly provide the support for a vacation state of mind. It is possible to create mini-vacations in our lives that serve to refresh and renew. By the time I got home this morning from my unexpected vacation, I felt a sense of calm and relaxation that led me to get more done, more easily than on those days when I rush and feel harried. So this is your vacation week. It may not be a week at the beach or even a trip to a special vacation spot, but it will be you naming experiences as vacation that will allow them to be pleasurable, renewing, and refreshing.

I know greater peace and happiness will be your travel companions as you take a vacation.

HOW TO DO IT

DAY 1: Take a vacation in your mind. Imagine your most relaxing scene:

- Close your eyes.
- Take five deep breaths, inhaling a sense of relaxation through your nose and exhaling through your mouth and into the earth, any undue stress or tension.
- Using the full resources of your imagination, create an image of your most relaxing scene.
- Seeing your most relaxing scene, notice the colors, hear the sounds, smell the fragrances, taste the tastes, and feel the feelings of your most relaxing scene. With a clear sense of this scene filling your being step into your most relaxing scene. Experience your most relaxing scene. (Do this for thirty to sixty seconds.)
- Experience a sense of vitality and renewal.
- Take a deep breath and relax your focus.
- Focus your attention on your breath, inhaling and exhaling three times.
- At your own speed, gently open your eyes, feeling wide awake, better than before, alert and fully connected with yourself and prepared for your day.

Use this technique in the morning, evening, and any time during the day that you need a vacation. Practice it daily, and your most relaxing scene will be available as a natural resource that pops into your mind, reminding you that you can always take a vacation in your mind. Remember, our being doesn't know the difference between being in far-off lands on a well-planned vacation or using our imagination to imagine a vacation.

DAY 2: Turn your lunch hour into vacation time today. If it's a nice day, go to a nearby park or new café with outdoor seating and imagine you are on an avenue in Paris enjoying people watching. If you love art and there is a nearby museum, go in and enjoy one great work of art that makes your heart sing. Use you imagination to turn your lunch hour into a glorious vacation. I used to meet my husband at his office in the midst of a busy day, and we'd go off for a forty-five-minute picnic. We'd find a grassy spot, put down a blanket, and enjoy what felt like a leisurely vacation lunch in the midst of our workday. (It's good to make a rule that there be no talk of work, kids, or home repairs during this vacation!)

DAY 3: Plan a vacation. Search the internet, get information, and plan a dream vacation. It may be as simple as a weekend in a nearby bed and breakfast to get a rest from your daily routine, or it may be a month-long trip you have desired for years. Dream it, see it, and take action to live it.

DAY 4: Take a pampering vacation today. Go for a manicure and pedicure and luxuriate in the pampering. Get a massage. When you work out at the gym, give yourself some extra time to use the sauna or steam room. When the kids have gone to bed or you have finished everything you have to do for the day, take a hot bath, using bubbles, your favorite oils, or a special soap. Light candles and turn off the lights, turn the phone ringer off, and feel the water against your body washing tension down the drain.

DAY 5: Approach your day as if you are on a vacation day, even if you are going to work, the supermarket, picking up the kids, seeing friends, and so forth. Do all your activities as though they are part of your vacation. If you ride public transportation, pretend this is the first time you have been on this bus route. Ask for directions as if you were on the Underground in London for the first time. If you drive, either take a new route, or actually look at where you are as you drive along this road you usually travel on automatic. Allow the spirit of vacation to be the filter, the glasses through which you see and experience your day.

DAY 6: Go someplace in your city or town where you have never been before. It may be an ethnic restaurant. Find out the specialty of the house, and order it as though you are a visitor in this new land. If you don't like it, you don't have to finish eating it, but you do have to acknowledge your willingness to be open to new experiences on your vacation. Go to a neighborhood you have never been to or haven't been to in a long time. Enjoy your vacation right where you live.

DAY 7: Write your reflections about your vacation week.

- What did you learn?
- How can you have more vacation time in your life?
- What if everyday was a vacation day, how would you approach it? Do it and allow peace and happiness to be a regular traveling companion.

week 36:
Eat Dessert First

Save the good stuff for last? Whose idea was that?

—SR

Eating dessert first is about having the good stuff first. Don't save it for a rainy day. Don't wait until tomorrow. Don't wait until you are the right weight, until your nails are the perfect length, until every issue in your life is worked out, until you have the right amount of money in the bank. Do it now. Many people spend their lives waiting, waiting to get married, waiting to finish school, waiting to have kids, waiting until their children are grown, waiting until they retire . . . waiting, waiting, waiting. All we have is now. The past is over, and the future lives in our imagination. Now is the precious present, a gift that contains all the power that ever was and ever will be. It is up to us to savor and delight in the present moment, to approach our life as a glorious magnificent buffet, and to reach for and enjoy the feast before us. So this week, eat dessert first and as you eat it, enjoy it; truly, this is the recipe for peace and happiness.

HOW TO DO IT

DAY 1: Today literally eat dessert first. Begin your meal with dessert. And if you are truly bold, have a meal of dessert only. Think about what dessert is for you. Don't limit it to cake, sweets, or ice cream. What is something you would love to eat? Something that makes you salivate simply by imagining it. And as you eat dessert first, enjoy it. If you notice you are making deals with yourself about the diet you'll begin tomorrow. Stop it. Enjoy now. This is not about stuffing yourself and bingeing. This is about savoring, delighting, enjoying, and allowing.

DAY 2: Think of something you have always wanted to do but didn't think you had the time, the money, or the know-how. Begin it today. If it's a trip you want to take, get information about it, call a travel agent, check the internet, mark it on your calendar. If it's a business you want to begin, see it as accomplished and take a step toward doing it. Bite into this dessert. If it's a relationship you desire, start by enjoying your life today and *seeing* what you want. When you see loving relationships, enjoy the pleasure of seeing what is possible and know it is on the menu of your life as well. Today choose the dessert you truly desire.

DAY 3: As you approach each activity of your day, consciously focus your attention on the *dessert* of the activity. As you get up and get ready for work, focus on how delicious it is to begin a new day. As you enter the supermarket, delight in the opportunity to choose a variety of items to make a tasty meal for yourself. As you walk to your weekly department meeting, smile as you think about this opportunity to share your ideas. As you step into each segment of your life, intend to have dessert.

DAY 4: Cook, bake, or prepare a great dessert. This may be an old favorite that brings loving memories to mind, it may be something you always wanted to make, or it may be an old family recipe that fills your house with mouth-watering aromas. Yum.

DAY 5: Invite friends and/or family for dinner and serve dessert first. Share your thoughts about having dessert first and let each person present know how he or she is dessert in your life.

DAY 6: Give a dessert to someone whom you'd like to appreciate with a treat. Leave a special cookie for your mail carrier, give the receptionist in your office his favorite sweet, or put a special dessert in your child's lunch box. Place a treat on your wife's pillow. Remember, what makes this dessert special is the love you put into it. So as you get it, prepare it, deliver it, do it all with love.

DAY 7: Write your reflections on eating dessert first.

- How can you keep this idea live in your daily life?
- What did you learn?

When you finish writing, eat dessert first!

WEEK 37:
Massage

*If you "don't have time" for a massage, you may be the one
who needs it the most.*

—LAHEY CLINIC, CANADA

Massage is a glorious form of touch that releases tension, fosters a deeper connection with our body, and offers the nourishment of loving touch. Often in our daily life there are many taboos about touch. The danger of accusations of sexual harassment stops us from reaching out and massaging a coworker's shoulders in the midst of a stressful work day. We sometimes hold back from asking for a massage for fear that we will be misunderstood and it will be assumed that this is actually a sexual innuendo. Sometimes when we are receiving a massage we are shy about saying harder, or softer; and when we are giving a massage, we question our competence. For these reasons massage is often seen a something outside of everyday activities. While a massage is definitely special, when it is incorporated into our daily experience, our well-being surges and peace and happiness abound.

While there are many different kinds of massage, for which people attend school and are licensed, even without receiving your license you can benefit both from receiving and giving a massage to a family member or friend. I often think of the stories I read in college psychology classes about the importance of touch for infant orphans. Studies were reported that demonstrated that orphaned infants who received only minimal touch would not grow and develop normally and would sometimes die. They were starved for touch. As adults we continue to have the same needs for physical connection. Massage is a form of touch that provides for this connection and soothes our body. It is a chance to move outside of our heads and feel with our magnificent sensing system, our bodies. When we experience a regular connection with our bodies, we are better able to use the guidance system of our physical sensations to indicate whether we are in heaven or hell.

This week give and receive massage and notice the impact on being peace and happiness from this simple act of touch.

HOW TO DO IT

DAY 1: Give your feet a massage today. Get some special oil, some foot massage lotion, or use some body oil you have in the house, and lovingly massage your feet. Imagine these are the feet of your beloved (aren't they?) and you are thanking them for all they do for you. Our feet carry us around all day, bearing the full weight of our bodies, sometimes squeezed into shoes that look better than they feel! Massage each toe, feel it, look at it. You may even say the toes poem from your childhood: this little piggy went to market, and so on. Notice what your skin feels like, where is it soft and smooth, where is it rough. Savor this glorious touch, and then move on to your next foot. To get the full benefit of this, do it in silence or with some relaxing music on so you can focus your attention on giving and receiving this loving massage. Spend a minimum of ten minutes on each foot. When you are finished massaging, put on a pair of cotton socks. Notice how your feet feel and how *you* feel.

DAY 2: Make an appointment for a massage for this week. If this is something you do regularly, make an appointment for a different kind of massage than usual. If this is something you have never done before, ask family and friends for their suggestions or call a spa or yoga center in your area for information and help in choosing what kind of massage to get and where to get it. You may also do a search on the internet to get descriptions of different kinds of massage (some forms of massage are: Swedish, Shiatsu, Reflexology, Sports, Trager, and so forth).

Sign up for a massage class. There are classes for individuals and couples. Check your local YMCA or community education programs as well as yoga centers to get information about massage classes in your area.

Go to your local library or bookstore and get a book and/or video on massage. Watch it, and then do it.

DAY 3: Give and receive three shoulder massages today. Ask family, friends, or coworkers if they'd be open to a shoulder massage trade. This can be as short as two minutes each, standing up; or longer with the receiver sitting down and the giver standing behind the receiver. When you are the giver ask the receiver to let you know what feels good, if he or she wants it harder or softer, higher or lower. It is also helpful to be silent other than for feedback. As the giver, allow yourself to feel what you are doing. I have found that when I allow the silence, I can often sense where to massage. When you finish giving the shoulder massage, shake the energy out of your hands. When you are the receiver, you may want to experiment with feeling what harder and softer feel like. Trust the cues of your body to let you know what feels good.

Be aware that if you have not experienced regular bodywork, you may be more sensitive than you expected. Our bodies hold our tension and the dramas of our past. Sometimes when we are touched, a sore spot that has been tight for years or months will be very sensitive to touch. The shoulder massages you are exchanging today are for relaxation.

Often when I lead Stress Management Workshops in corporate settings I will end the workshop with the participants making a circle and massaging the shoulders of the person in front of them, first asking for permission to touch, and then turning around and massaging the person who just massaged them. There is often laughter, since it is so different from business as usual in the workplace, as well as sighs of pleasant feelings.

DAY 4: Get a quick massage today. There are many nail salons that offer short shoulder and neck massages for men and women (ten minutes for ten dollars). Some cities and malls also have walk-in massages for shoulders and necks for a dollar per minute. I know of some organizations providing this kind of massage as part of their employee wellness programs. Sometimes the organization pays, sometimes the employees pay, and sometimes they split the fee. If you're a boss or own a business, you may want to look into this as an idea for a treat for your employees one day, once a week, once a month, or during a particularly stressful time at work.

DAY 5: When you get out of the shower or bath today, massage your body with oil or body lotion. So often we automatically get out of the shower or bath, get dried, possibly use body lotion, get dressed, and move on to our next activity. Today, if you have the radio turned on to the news, turn it off, or if the TV is hooking your attention, turn it off, and in silence massage your body. Feel what your skin feels like on different parts of your body. Know that the oil or moisturizing lotion you are using combined with your loving touch is nourishing your body. Did you know that your skin is your largest organ? It is exposed to heat and cold and all different types of fabrics, so honor it today, pay attention to it, nourish it as you massage it slowly and carefully.

DAY 6: Trade a massage with a family member or friend. It may be a full body massage, a foot massage, back and shoulders—you decide.

DAY 7: Write your reflections on massage.

- What did you learn this week focusing on massage?
- What was your experience giving? Receiving?
- How did massage contribute to peace and happiness?
- How can you incorporate massage into your life?

week 38:
Have a New Thought

Thoughts held in mind, manifest over time.
—ERNEST HOLMES

Having a new thought is about consciously choosing where you put your attention. Since our thoughts are the seeds of the life we create and live, what we think is very important. Often people are asleep to their thoughts, both the ones that run like a continuous tape in their heads as well as the ones that they articulate. Have you ever looked at yourself in the mirror in the morning and thought with conviction, "I look awful"? That is a powerful example of self-abuse, and it is the perfect time to have a new thought. This week your practice is two-fold:

1. Become aware of your thoughts. It is a daunting task to pay attention to each and every thought. A simple approach is to pay attention to your feelings. When you are feeling good, check in with yourself and notice your thoughts. When you are feeling bad, victimized, unworthy, journeying on a one-way ticket to hell, ask yourself, "What am I thinking right now that is creating an experience of hell for me?"
2. Have a new thought when your thoughts are abusive and judgmental of yourself or others.

HOW TO DO IT

DAY 1: Check in with yourself throughout the day and listen to your thoughts. When you wake up in the morning, what are your first thoughts? When you are eating, what are you telling yourself? When you look at yourself in the mirror, what are your thoughts? As you travel to work, when you are with your spouse, friends, lover, coworkers, when you are waiting for the elevator, what are the thoughts you feed yourself? Do these thoughts support peace and happiness? If not, have a new thought.

DAY 2: Write down your beliefs. Remember, beliefs are thought habits, thoughts you have thought repeatedly, so you think they are true. What are your beliefs about yourself, love, romance, work, family, health, finances, peace on Earth, God, and so forth? Are your beliefs aligned with peace and happiness? If not, have a new thought.

Listening to the song by Savage Garden called "I Believe" on their *Affirmation* CD is helpful in preparing for this exercise.

DAY 3: Listen to yourself as you speak. Do your words support peace and happiness, or are they abusive and judgmental? If they are abusive and judgmental, change them right then and there.

DAY 4: Appreciate yourself for waking up and noticing your thoughts and words. It is important that you be self-accepting; otherwise you are reinforcing abusive and judgmental behavior. Whenever you notice your thoughts throughout the day, give yourself a pat on the back for your enhanced awareness.

DAY 5: Make a list of thoughts that support peace and happiness and the life that you want to live. Some of the thoughts on my list are:

- I am love.
- Health and well-being are my daily experience.
- Everything I eat turns to health and beauty.
- I am abundant and prosperous.
- I am sexy and sensual.
- I am successful in my work.
- Everyone is an expression of God.

From this list make signs to put around your home, office, and car as reminders of the thoughts you want to fill your life with, the thoughts you want to think often enough to create a new set of beliefs.

DAY 6: Since human beings are natural storytellers, much of the angst we experience is based on the stories we make up about the circumstances we experience. When we realize we have the power to make up new stories, we can transform our lives in the moment. I remember many years ago, when I participated in an est workshop, human beings were described as meaning-making machines. Today, play with making up multiple stories about the circumstance you experience. For instance, if your boss stops by your desk and asks you to come into her office, here are some possible stories/thoughts you can have about it:

- Oh, she must want to compliment me on the project I just completed.
- There must be something important she wants to tell me.

- I wonder what I did wrong.
- Oh good, this will give me a chance to thank her for being flexible with my work schedule the past two days.

Knowing that we make up the stories and choose our thoughts, choose to focus on thoughts that are supportive of heaven rather than falling into the trap of anticipating hell. This technique can also be applied to making up a new story about your past!

DAY 7: Write your reflections on having new thoughts.

- What did you notice about your thoughts?
- What was the impact on your experience when you had a new thought?
- How did having a new thought contribute to your peace and happiness?

The greatest discovery of our generation is that a human being can alter his life by altering his attitudes.

—WILLIAM JAMES

week 39:
Live Abundantly

Life is a banquet and most people are starving.
—FROM *AUNTIE MAME*

Living abundantly begins with your point of view. So often we think that our abundance will be determined by the material possessions we have. We will be abundant when we have a new car, new house, newer computer, or a salary increase. Then we get a new car, a new house, a newer computer, and a salary increase, and rather than feeling prosperous and abundant, all we notice is our increased monthly bills, or we worry that these new things that we desired will break down or won't last. In the midst of having received our heart's desire, our consciousness continues to focus on lack. Each time a new desire surfaces, instead of greeting it with open arms and faith in our creative ability, we get lost in the dissatisfaction of what is.

In order to live abundantly we must have an inner experience of abundance, prosperity, peace, and happiness that is independent of the things we have. I recently saw a quote that captures this idea: "If you want to make more money then you have to decide to be worth more." It highlights that our experience of abundance and prosperity begins in our consciousness.

As you read this, you may notice a voice within you saying, "Then why are people starving? Why do some people have more than others?" A usual way to address questions like this is to talk about power, government, economics, and the unfairness of the world, and about the powerful who take advantage of the weak, business executives who have inside information and sell their stock at huge profits before the general public gets the information. When you think about these situations, it's easy to rely on the tried-and-true beliefs about the world being unfair, or that you can't trust government or the wealthy, or that people are greedy. When you focus on lack, unfairness, and greed in the world rather than on abundance, your thoughts contribute to this lack. It is easy to find evidence of lack if that is your point of view. It is *just* as easy to see evidence of abundance if that is your lens of perception. This is not about denying the full range of expressions of creation on earth; it is about using your power to focus your attention on the abundant world you desire and believing that your creative power is real. All we actually have control over is what we think and where we put our attention. Whether or not you believe this, try acting as if it is true, and notice the change in your personal world and in how you see the global community when you focus your attention on living abundantly.

Abundance and Me

My life is abundant. From the outside it has always looked that way. For many years it didn't seem that way to me. I focused on what I didn't have and worried that I wouldn't get what I really wanted. When I got it, there was always something else to want, so I didn't really enjoy anything I'd gotten. In 1997, from the outside, my life looked enviable. I was married to a local celebrity in my high-profile community. I was part of a large family. I lived in a house with a view of majestic sunsets on the bay. I drove a fire-engine red sports car. I had a lucrative consulting practice, and I made my own hours. I traveled first-class on airplanes, stayed in the best hotels in the world, and had dinner with celebrities. I wore a big diamond ring and got a mink coat for a Valentine's Day gift. My bills were paid. I knew interesting people and had loving friends. A housekeeper kept my house. My office was a beautiful sanctuary.

But I was miserable, as nothing was enough for me. I was angry, and I blamed my husband, my stepkids, and mostly myself for not being pretty enough, sexy enough, thin enough, good enough, and loveable enough. My life collapsed. My husband decided to divorce me and immediately begin a new relationship. I was devastated. I decided to approach this crisis as though I had been diagnosed with a terminal illness. I knew that this would be an inside job. If I didn't change the programming in me, no matter what I did to the outside, there would be no sustaining change. It was time for me to walk my talk and put all the ideas and skills I had taught others fully into practice. With the help of wonderful therapists, teachers, friends, and family, I reinvented myself. I did it by making up a new story about me and the world in which I live: "I Am a Loved and Loving Child of a Loving Universe."

Today I see all life through the eyes of wonder. When I hear about suffering, I send prayers of love to that part of the world, and I am grateful for reminders that life is precious and that I need to honor today. This summer many children throughout the country have been abducted, some killed, some safely returned home. I asked myself, "Okay, how do you view this?" I thought, "I am grateful to be reminded that children are precious and to honor the children in my life and the child that lives within each and everyone of us."

Abundance is looking through rose-colored glasses. Pollyanna is a good role model. Isn't it time to give them a try?

—SR

HOW TO DO IT

Resource

~ *The Abundance Book* by John Randolph Price, Carlsbad, CA: Hay House, 1996.

DAY 1: Complete the following statement as fully as possible: An abundant person believes: _____.

After you have written your list, make sure that each item supports what an abundant person is, rather than what she or he is not. Some examples are:

- An abundant person trusts in the universe to support his desires, rather than, an abundant person doesn't worry about his desires being met.
- An abundant person acknowledges accomplishments, rather than, an abundant person doesn't focus on what is not working.

Now rewrite the list in the first person:

- I trust the universe to support my desires.
- I easily acknowledge my accomplishments each step of the way.

Read this list aloud each morning when you wake up, at night before you go to sleep, and whenever your personal programming needs an abundance zap. When you start to read it, first say your intention: "I am installing my new and improved abundance programming."

DAY 2: Make a list of the riches in your life right now. If you want abundance in the future, the starting place is seeing abundance NOW, in your present. Some items on my list are:

- Loving friendships
- Great car
- Health
- Satisfying work
- Beautiful hair
- Comfortable bed
- Beautiful home
- Great CDs to listen to
- My dream soulmate
- Strong muscles
- Good teeth
- Well-stocked cupboards
- Supportive community

Be playful with this list and read it when you need to be reminded of the abundance in your life.

DAY 3: Buy yourself something special today. This is not about cost. This is about buying something that symbolizes abundance in your life. It may be a new CD you want but didn't think you should spend the money, a bouquet of flowers, or a single rose. You may order the sandwich that you really want but you usually don't order because it is three dollars more than the other sandwiches on the menu. Act as if you are abundant today and be abundant today.

DAY 4: Be generous. True generosity, with no strings attached, expecting nothing in return, and no score keeping is a direct expression of abundance. Be generous with your time and skills by volunteering for something you believe in; leave an extra tip for a waiter; give away thank-yous. Go through your closet and gather up things you don't wear or use and donate them to a homeless shelter.

DAY 5: Experiment with tithing. There is a universal law of tenfold return. This means that when you give freely your return is tenfold. You don't give to get the return, you give freely and what you give flows back to you tenfold. Particularly in terms of money, many of us think the law of attraction doesn't apply here. It does. Money is simply energy, and when we allow the energy to flow through us, then money and resources continue to flow to us. When we stop the flow out of fear, anxiety, and worry, the flow stops. During the next six months, experiment. Whenever you get money, before you pay any bill, take ten percent of that and give it to something you believe in. What is most important is that you give with an open heart.

DAY 6: Have a conversation with five people about abundance. Share your ideas about an abundant life starting with abundant thoughts.

DAY 7: Write your reflections on abundance.

- What did you learn about your relationship with abundance this week?
- How does your experience with abundance relate to peace and happiness?
- What are the most powerful thoughts for you to believe in order for you to be abundant?

week 40:
Hug

Heartfelt
Unconditional
Gratitude

—SUSAN IVORY

Hugs are an expression of love and support. Sometimes you give a hug when you have an irresistible urge of delight and love that you want to express physically. Other hugs are a warm, caring embrace that let the people you are hugging know that you are there for them, that they are not alone. And some hugs are expressions of passion, a sensual, sexual embrace. We live in a culture that has taboos about touching and hugging. We can hug family and close friends, but in the workplace it may not be okay to hug a coworker unless there is a good reason for it, such as their going-away party! Sometimes we hold back from hugging because we worry about what the other person will think. Sometimes we hold back because we don't want to intrude, and sometimes we hold back simply from lack of hugging practice. Sometimes we don't ask for a hug because we are afraid of being rejected, or we worry about imposing on someone, or we're concerned that this physical contact may be misinterpreted. Hugs are a natural part of peace and happiness. They say, "I love you; I care for you; I'm here for you." This week, HUG—when you feel the urge to ask for a hug, ask for it and receive it. When you feel the urge to give a hug, give it.

HOW TO DO IT

RESOURCE

~ Georgia Girl Hugs website: *www. gagirl.com/hugs/hug.html.*

DAY 1: Give ten hugs today. Notice how you hug. Do you get right in there and allow yourself to fully give and receive? Do you hold back, unsure of the "right way" to do this? Whom is it easy for you to hug, and whom are you hesitant to hug?

DAY 2: Ask for and receive ten hugs today. Notice what this experience is like for you. What did you learn about yourself and hugging?

DAY 3: Send a long-distance hug to a loved one. You may call her on the phone with an "I love you" message. You may send an email and tell him to take a moment to feel the hug you have enclosed in the email. Be creative and let the person know that you are sending a hug their way.

DAY 4: Write a poem, essay, or song about hugs.

DAY 5: Hug yourself five times today. You can actually wrap your arms around yourself and allow yourself to feel you embracing you. Hug yourself by taking care of you. If you are blue and need a hug of encouragement, rent your favorite movie and feel it hugging you as you snuggle up and watch it. If you are delighted with yourself, hug your fingernails with glittery nail polish. Be creative in hugging yourself today.

DAY 6: Write about what holds you back from giving, asking for, and receiving hugs. What are new thoughts you can have that would make this expression of love easier for you? If hugs are a challenge for you, imagine that you are a person who easily gives and receives hugs and identify thoughts that make hugging easy. Create a new story about you being the most fabulous hugger on earth. With three people today, be the most fabulous hugger on earth.

DAY 7: Write about your experience of asking for, receiving, and giving hugs.

- What did you learn about yourself?
- How can you spread hugs around?

We need 4 hugs a day for survival. We need 8 hugs a day for maintenance. We need 12 hugs a day for growth.

—VIRGINIA SATIR

week 41:
Detach and Let Go

In our willingness to step into the unknown, the field of all possibilities, we surrender ourselves to the creative mind that orchestrates the dance of the universe.

—Deepak Chopra

Detaching and letting go is how we release from the past, unhook from unsatisfying habits of thought and behavior, and live life fully in the precious present. Many of us begin each new day loaded down with emotional baggage, limiting beliefs, and expectations based on past circumstances that we define as truth. These attachments to circumstances, relationships, addictions, and patterns of thought and behavior are often experienced as a lifetime prison sentence with occasional moments off for good behavior. As human beings, we tend to follow the path of least resistance in our thoughts and actions, which means we repeat patterns and habits on automatic, without thinking, in a sleep state even though our eyes are wide open. To create a new pattern requires the conscious focus of our attention on how we feel and what we think, say, and do. To focus our attention requires the energy of our personal power. The paradox is that our energy is already being used to hold the old patterns and habits in place. It is as though we are caught in a spider's web, and to detach and let go, we have to free ourselves from each thread and cable of the web. Sometimes, we can go right to the core thread, which is some variation of "I am not enough," or "I'm not okay." Detach from that idea, and automatically let go of patterns and behaviors that were dependent on that core idea for their nourishment and survival. This week, as you detach and let go, you are saying, YES to a deeper and fuller experience of personal freedom, and isn't that what peace and happiness is?

CAUTION: This is not the time to judge and beat yourself up for your limiting beliefs and lousy habits. Don't use this week's exercises to prove to yourself that since you are still stuck, you will always be stuck. Instead, enjoy this opportunity to free your energy, make conscious choices, detach, and let go.

HOW TO DO IT

DAY 1: Today is the day to detach and let go of stuff. You may choose your in-box at the office, your closet, your medicine cabinet, or your underwear drawer. Choose something that when you see it, you feel overwhelmed by the clutter and burdened by the disorganization. Clean it out. Let go of stuff. Notice the infusion of energy you feel when you are finished. Close the drawer, leave the room, and the next time you open the drawer or enter the room, feel a greater lightness filling your being. If you notice, rather than feeling the freedom of letting go, you are being abusive to yourself for waiting so long to do this, STOP IT. You did it today, and this counts. The past is over, so let it go.

DAY 2: Let go of one person or situation in your life. For instance, if you're still angry at your former spouse, from whom you've been divorced for four years, let go of this anger. If you have wanted to lose weight for a long time and every diet you go on lasts no longer than one week, let go of the self-hate cycle. If your financial situation keeps you up at night with worry, find ways to move through the problem. If all of these apply to you, for the sake of this exercise, choose only one to begin with, or you'll be in such a quandary about which one to choose that you'll exhaust yourself without doing the exercise! Once you've chosen a practice situation:

- Sit comfortably.
- Close your eyes.
- Focus on your breath.
- Take three full deep breaths. Breathe in through your nose a sense of calming relaxation and exhale fully and deeply through your mouth, allowing yourself to relax fully into the support of the chair you are sitting on.
- Using the full resources of your imagination, see yourself attached by a thread or a cable to the situation or person worrying you, draining your energy.
- Take a pair of scissors or metal cable cutters, and cut the attachment from where it is connected to your body.
- When you cut the thread of connection, see the situation or person, like a helium balloon that has been released, begin to disappear from your sight as it drifts up and away getting smaller and smaller until it is gone.

- Feel lightness in your being and more energy.
- Gently open your eyes, feeling better than before.

Use this technique any time you are attached to something as a way of detaching and letting go. By freeing up your energy from your connection to your worry and fear, you have more energy to focus your attention on what you do want to create in the present moment. If the same situation pops into your mind at another time, it doesn't mean that this technique doesn't work. It is simply a reminder to detach again, and again and again and again, if necessary. Old habits sometimes like to stick around!

DAY 3: Use the "Oops technique." Anytime you notice you are caught in a web of abusive and judgmental thoughts about yourself or others, simply say aloud or to yourself, "Oops," and get on a new train of thought. Approach this as though you have simply made a wrong turn, and all you do is say, "Oops," before you get back on track with thoughts that enhance your peace and happiness.

DAY 4: Practice detaching and letting go of habits today by doing things differently. This is actually practice in increasing your flexibility, something we need when we let go. If you usually brush your teeth with your right hand, use your left. Hold the phone to your other ear. Put your watch on your other wrist. Use your nondominant hand to hold a spoon. Use the elliptical trainer at the gym rather than the treadmill. Put a sock on your left foot first. Be creative. You will probably notice you feel odd when you make these changes. This is ordinary, because when we detach and let go of habits we are used to, the new behavior feels awkward. If you continue to do some of these changes regularly for the next month you will notice you have created a new habit that feels familiar. Some of them will become new habits in only a few days!

DAY 5: Use your feelings as your guidance system to let you know when you are attached to something. Whenever you are consumed by feelings of unhappiness, sadness, anger, loneliness, or any feelings that create a personal hell, this is a pretty good indicator you are attached to an idea that is draining your energy. When you notice any of these feelings today, use the "Oops technique" and focus your attention on a new thought that feels satisfying. This doesn't mean you will never have an unhappy feeling again. It means you can use your feelings as your guidance system and make choices about where you continue to focus your attention. Recently, I was missing Mom, who died in December, 2001 and I noticed I was beginning to settle into feeling miserable. There was a domino effect of all these other situations and circumstances I felt blue about. I noticed I was allowing my sadness to take me on a roller-coaster ride. I took a deep breath and began having a conversation, in my mind, with Mom. Within minutes I had a smile on my face remembering special times with her. I felt my sadness and used it to move into a deeper experience of Mom's presence.

DAY 6: On one side of a page make a list of thoughts and behaviors you have been attached to that do not serve you. When you have completed that side of the page, go back to the first item and beside it, write a new thought or behavior that is more supportive of peace and happiness. Here are some examples:

I'm never gonna loose this weight.	My body is beautiful, healthy, and fit.
I'll be single forever.	I'm in a loving relationship.
My kids never listen to me.	I love my relationship with my kids.
I get no recognition at work.	I feel good about the job I do.

This is practice in changing your programming, detaching and letting go of thoughts that reinforce what you don't want, and creating a new script, which will then direct your eyes to seeing your experience from a new point of view. Be playful. Remember you are the dream and the dreamer of your life!

DAY 7: Write a poem about detaching and letting go. Write your reflections on detaching and letting go.

- What did you learn?
- How can you use the detaching and letting go techniques in your daily life?

We must learn to let go, to give up, to make room for the things we have prayed for and desired.
—CHARLES FILLMORE

week 42:
Smile

*Sometimes your joy is the source of your smile, but sometimes
your smile can be the source of your joy.*
—THICH NHAT HANH

Smiling is a simple, magical gesture that expresses peace and happiness. It is a gift we can easily give. When we give it away to others, we clearly get the benefit of the energy of the smile moving through us. I remember hearing on a stress management video many years ago that it takes seventeen muscles to smile and forty-three to frown. So it involves much less effort than a scowl, and in the words of a Ziggy cartoon, "A SMILE is a facelift that's in everyone's price range!!"

I have noticed the power of a smile to change my experience in the moment. I have recently returned to practicing yoga. Usually once or twice during our class, the instructor, Ani Kalfayan, will say, "Turn up the corners of your mouth. Yoga is meant to be joyful." I follow her instructions, and immediately I experience a lightness of being. As I do this, my eyes are usually closed, and I feel the power of my smile embracing me. I have also noticed the power of a smile when I am paying a cashier. Words may not even be exchanged and magic immediately happens. A connection is made, and the present moment becomes a precious present. I am also aware that I have another smile. It's the sourpuss smile, and behind this smile a judge is holding court, doling out judgments, and communicating to others what I may be thinking I am hiding.

This week, get to know your smiles and use your smiles to share your love and be a gateway to moving your experience from sad to glad. Play and smile and imagine all the peace and happiness we would experience each and every day if we let a smile lead our way.

HOW TO DO IT

DAY 1: Give away fifty smiles today. As a reminder, write SMILE in bright letters on your calendar, on Post-Its you put around your house, car, and workplace. Put it on your screen saver, as a reminder message on your Palm Pilot; leave yourself a Voicemail message that says, SMILE.

DAY 2: Smile to yourself fifty times today. When you are walking down the street and you notice a neutral expression or a frown on your face, SMILE. While you're in the shower, SMILE.

DAY 3: Make a list of all the things and memories that make you smile when you think about them. Post the list somewhere you can see it, and five times today look at the list, choose an item from your list, and put your attention on it, feeling a smile fill your being. This is a powerful practice of consciously choosing where to focus your attention. The more practice we have, the more easily we can access happy thoughts when drama thoughts are flirting with us. You are strengthening your happy thoughts muscle today.

DAY 4: Every time you look in a mirror today, smile at yourself. A smile that says, "I'm glad to see you," "You're one handsome dude," "You're beautiful," "I'm beautiful."

DAY 5: Do a search of the web for "smile quotes." Find ones that make you smile. Copy them, put them somewhere you can see them, and put one in the bottom of your sock drawer so it pops out at you one day at the most perfect time.

DAY 6: Think of three people you know who put a smile on your face and write them a note telling them.

DAY 7: Write your reflections on smiling.

- What did you learn about smiling this week?
- How do you feel when you smile?
- How can you remember to make smiles part of your daily life?

What sunshine is to flowers, smiles are to humanity. These are but trifles, to be sure; but, scattered along life's pathway, the good they do is inconceivable.

—JOSEPH ADDISON

If you have only one smile in you, give it to the people you love. Don't be surly at home, then go out in the street and start grinning "Good morning" at total strangers.

—MAYA ANGELOU

Seize the moment, be here now.
Make lemonade out of lemons.
Imagine Peace and Happiness.
Live your dreams.
Eat dessert first.

      —SR

week 43:
Spend Time with a Friend

*Each friend represents a world in us, a world possibly not born
until they arrive, and it is only by this meeting that a new
world is born.*

—Anaïs Nin

Spending time with a friend is a gift of love we give ourselves. Friends are treasures. They giggle with us, they remind us of who we are, and they are mirrors reflecting our radiance. They are shoulders to cry on, buddies to do things with, and lifelines when the road gets rough. Spending time with a friend is a vital root of peace and happiness. This week, cultivate this treasure of life by spending time with a friend.

HOW TO DO IT

DAY 1: Spend time with a friend today. Call a friend on the spur of the moment and make plans to meet for lunch, or settle in on the couch with the phone and talk with your best friend who lives in another part of the country. Connect with a friend today.

DAY 2: Send a card to a friend today that expresses your love and care for this special being in your life.

DAY 3: Do a friendship inventory:

- Who are the friends who you can call anytime, day or night, when you need a shoulder to cry on?
- Who are the friends you can count on to confront you, the one's who remind you that you have been singing that tune for many months now, and ask how they can help you to move on?
- Who are the friends you enjoy doing things with?
- Who are the friends who tell you what they think, not simply what they think you want to hear?
- Who are the friends to share adventures with?
- Who are the friends you allow yourself to be vulnerable with, the ones you call late at night when you are feeling alone, the ones you are eager to share the good news with?

After you have completed your inventory, notice what this tells you. Any changes you want to make? Make them!

DAY 4: Make a friendship celebration date with a friend or group of friends. This is a day to celebrate your friendship. You may go out and get a manicure together, go to your favorite sports event, eat at your favorite restaurant, share a meal you've cooked together in one of your homes. Make sure you use some of your time together to express and acknowledge that this time together is a celebration of your friendship.

DAY 5: Get in touch with an old friend whom you have wondered about. Call the last phone number you have for her, send a note to his last address, or search an internet directory. If none of that works, have a conversation with her in your mind, let him know that you are thinking of him and that you'd love the opportunity to talk with him. Have faith that this communication is getting to her.

I have two childhood friends whom I sought out in my consciousness for many years. They would pop into my mind, and I felt I was putting a call out into the universe for them. In each case, a few years later they popped up, each at the most perfect time. One of them I am still in touch with. We first met when our mothers took us to the local park in our strollers when we were a few months old. I love this connection with someone who knew me way back when. The other friend and I stayed in touch briefly, and she shared her perception of me when we were teenagers. It was a powerful reminder that my perception of myself had been quite judgmental. She gave me a new, complimentary point of view.

DAY 6: Today be your best friend. Treat yourself as though you are a treasure. See yourself through the eyes of your best friend. Be gentle, be loving, be accepting, be your own best friend.

DAY 7: Write your reflections on spending time with a friend.

- What did you learn about friendship in your life?
- How do your friendships contribute to your peace and happiness?
- Are there any changes you want to make? Make them!

The greatest sweetener of human life is friendship.

—Joseph Addison

week 44:
Take a Risk

*And then the day came when the risk to remain tight in the
bud was more painful than the risk it took to blossom.*
—ANAÏS NIN

Taking a risk means stepping outside of everyday habits and con-sciously make choices that echo your heart song. Taking a risk is doing something in a different way, whether it is changing your thinking or taking a different action. It often opens the way to new possi-bilities and ultimately to a greater experience of peace and happiness. Sometimes, taking a risk means speaking up and voicing your point of view; other times a risk is remaining silent and listening. A risk may be to start a new business, to talk with your boss about a raise, to enroll in a class, to try out for a part with your local theater group. A risk may be to share your love with a loved one or to go to the gym even though you don't remember when you last exercised. A risk is to get a new haircut, or to wear the clothes you have only tried on in the privacy of your room. A risk may be to go on a trip by yourself, or to ask for help.

Life is filled with opportunities to be fully alive, to live our heart's desire. It is up to us to take the action, take the risk, and feel the personal freedom we have access to when we say, "Yes." So this week, take a risk, and if you experience fear or feel paralyzed, take a deep breath and do it anyway. Keep in mind that this is not about being a daredevil. This is about listening to the message of your heart and responding with a resounding, YES.

HOW TO DO IT

DAY 1: In the words of Robert Frost, take the road less traveled today. Take a risk. Get a new haircut. Say, "I love you" aloud. Sign up at the gym. Find out about that investment you have been wondering about. Enroll in the comedy workshop you've daydreamed about.

DAY 2: Risk dreaming your big dream. Write down your heart's desire. If you knew you couldn't fail and that all the resources of the universe were available to you, what would you dare to dream? Would you be in a leading role on Broadway, or traveling the world, or be a physician, or be at home

when your kids are finished with school each day, or turning your grandmother's apple pie recipe into a successful business and donating a portion
of the profit to a cause you love? This is the dream to write down today. Go
for it. Dream big. Start your writing in the present tense with the following
sentence:

Today I am fully living my heart's desire, my big dream. I am:

DAY 3: Take a step to live your big dream today.

DAY 4: Create a virtual reality of your big dream and visualize it for sixty
seconds three times a day (today and every day). See yourself living your
dream. Use the full resources of your imagination as you live the virtual reality of your heart's desire. Be specific about where you are, what you are wearing, the sounds you hear, the tastes and fragrances of your heart's desire,
how you are feeling. Make sure to put yourself into the scene.

DAY 5: Risk expressing your love today. Allow every thought you think, every
word you say, and every action you take to be an expression of love. If, by
habit, you make a slip, simply ask yourself, "What would love do here?" and
get back on track.

DAY 6: Every time you get a nudge today to do an act of kindness, act on it.
If there is someone on the street asking you for money and even if you wonder
if she will simply use the money for a drink, give anyway. If you see some
trash on the street and are inclined to pick it up, bend down and pick it up.
If it seems as if the person in front of you at the supermarket needs some
help with their packages, offer to help.

DAY 7: Write a poem about your experience of taking a risk. Write what you
have learned about being a risk taker this week.

- How does taking risks enhance your experience of peace and
  happiness?
- How can you incorporate this point of view in your life so you risk
  expressing your love to yourself and those around you, every day?

I am always doing that which I cannot do, in order that I may
learn to do it.

   —PABLO PICASSO

week 45:
Go to the Movies

Movies are the most electrifying communications medium ever devised and the natural conduit for inspiring ourselves to look into the eternal issues of who we are and why we are here.

—STEPHEN SIMON

Going to the movies is a wonderful way to engage and connect with a story that can excite you, dazzle you, open your heart, remind you of the magnificence, as well as the destructiveness, of human beings. Movies are the modern-day version of gathering around the campfire and hearing stories. They are fairy tales, and rather than being passed on through an oral tradition, they invade our senses with surround sound and visual effects that at times seem to reach out to us in our seats. (Keep in mind that fairy tales are stories that speak to the soul's journey, and it is their deeper meaning that engages the soul in ways that are usually not immediately apparent.) On a big screen, stories are bigger than life and a slice of life, visual and auditory representations of thoughts that spring from the minds of people.

Movies can be a glorious escape from whatever circumstances we are in the midst of and can also touch us emotionally and wake us up from the daily drama of our own lives. Movies can surprise us and imbed images in our minds that capture our attention. Depending on what these images are, the road to fear or love is illuminated. Movies show us the full range of what is possible in terms of what the human mind can create and the experiences that human beings have in life. This week, use movies as a gateway to peace and happiness and allow them to open your eyes to what is possible. As you watch the movies and enjoy and reflect on their stories, remember that our lives are unfolding stories and that we are the screenwriter, the producer, the director, and the leading character in the movie of our lives. With that in mind, what movies would you like to watch to give you ideas for the movie of your life?

HOW TO DO IT

resources
_____

~ *The Force Is with You: Mystical Movie Messages That Inspire Our Lives* by
  Stephen Simon, Charlottesville, VA: Hampton Roads Publishing Co.,
  2002.
~ *Cinematherapy—The Girl's Guide to Movies for Every Mood* by Nancy
  Peske and Beverly West, New York: Dell Books, 1999.

DAY 1: Make a list of your all-time favorite movies and next to each one jot
down what is special about it to you. Is it a movie that makes you laugh out loud?
Are you inspired by it? Norman Cousins writes in his book, *Anatomy of an
Illness*, of the power of laughter in treating and curing a life-threatening
tissue disease he had. He watched Marx Brothers movies from his hospital
bed. In the midst of serious illness, movies provided the focus for him to
laugh, laugh, and laugh. Here are some of my favorites, with a brief description of why I like them:

- *The Matrix*—creating our experience
- *Where Dreams Come From*—the power of thought in creating our
  experience
- *Life As a House*—how peoples' lives are changed in the presence of love
- *Pay It Forward*—the power of each of us to change the world
- *Beauty and the Beast*—the power of love
- *Monsters, Inc.*—how our thoughts feed our fears
- *Forrest Gump*—being who you are and always doing your best
- *Dead Man Walking*—seeing everyone as an expression of God
- *Road to Perdition*—fathers and sons; the life-giving power of love and
  the destructive power of jealousy and envy
- *Monsoon Wedding*—the healing power of love
- *Resurrection*—fear of love and the healing power of love
- *Starman*—fear of the unknown
- *Keeping the Faith*—the power of faith
- *Rabbit Free Fence*—the desire to be free

DAY 2: Choose a movie from your list to rent and watch. Make yourself comfortable. Pop the popcorn and allow the movie to capture your attention.

DAY 3: Go to the movies and see a movie that you might not ordinarily see.
If you usually don't see movies with subtitles, treat yourself to one today; see

an animated movie or an action movie. Experiment and allow the movie to tell you its story without judging that this isn't the kind of movie you usually see.

DAY 4: Ask five people today what their three all-time favorite movies are and why. Then rent and watch one of them, or if it's playing in a theater near you, go and see it.

DAY 5: If you have home movies, watch some. Allow this trip down memory lane to remind you of times of your life. Many years after my husband, Byll, and I divorced, he sent me a video compilation of movies from the years we were married. It is something I treasure, a reminder of glorious times and adventures we had. Long after the ouch of the divorce had healed, what remained was reminders of good times. If by chance you are holding on to old pains, it is possible that seeing some videos of times you enjoyed can serve as a reminder that your past was also filled with happy times. If you don't have home movies to watch, journey through some photo albums of your life.

It is important to remember that we have the ability to experience greater personal freedom when we free ourselves from the drama of our past, the movie reel (real?) that runs in our minds about our personal stories. We have an opportunity to change our experience of our pasts by what we choose to remember and the story we tell ourselves about it. So choose to remember the scenes of life that are empowering, and forgive and put to rest the others.

DAY 6: Go to the movies today and allow memories of movie fun times to pop into your mind.

DAY 7: Write your reflections on going to the movies.

- How can you use this idea of going to the movies to enhance your experience of peace and happiness?
- Make a list of "Movies I Wanna See" and see them.

Is This Real?

My oldest sister, Ruth, often took me to the movies when I was a child. There were double features then and we would be in the theater for many hours. I remember often turning to her, tapping her on the arm, and whispering, "Is this really happening right now? Is this really going on in real life?" It took me quite a while to learn that the movie reel and real life were two different things. This continues to be helpful to me today when I remember that the stories of my life, my interpretations of events, are like a movie reel and that I can change those reels.

—SR

week 46:
Live Your Dreams

And the dreams that you dare to dream really do come true.
—From "Over The Rainbow,"
E.Y. Harburg & Harold Arlen

Living your dreams is a direct route to peace and happiness. Your dreams are your heart song, desires alive in you. Unfortunately, many of us are living our nightmare, waiting until tomorrow to live our dreams or trying to convince ourselves that our dreams are just that, dreams, not something real and possible in our lives. Yet it is through living our dreams that doors and windows open to a satisfying, fulfilling, and joyous life. It is through living our dreams that we truly honor our lives as a precious present.

Everything that exists in the world begins as a dream, an idea, a vision, a thought, whether it is a paperclip or a relationship, love or fear. Everything is created twice, first as a dream and then in our three-dimensional reality. We are dreamers and when we dream with our heart and follow that song, magic happens.

You have probably had experiences in your life when, in a spurt of inspiration, an idea, a dream, enters your consciousness fully formed. A vision of a new job, relationship, solution to a problem, or a new path to take. You feel a powerful surge of loving energy move through you as this desire, your heart song, captures your attention. In the moment, you decide to follow your dream. Then life happens and you begin to doubt the possibility of your dream. If you use these times of doubt as springboards to recommit to your dream, as time goes by, all sorts of support will present themselves. You will get the money to enroll in school, you will get the job you love, you will find venture capital for your new invention, you will create a deep loving relationship in your life. If, on the other hand, you allow the voice of fear to be the narrator of your dream, you will decide that your heart song, while a nice idea, is simply not going to happen. And with that decision, you stop breathing life into your dream.

Since we are dreamers anyway and we create our experience through an alchemical process that combines our thoughts, beliefs, and energy (our e-motion—energy in motion), we might as well dream the dreams and live the life that we truly desire. This week, take steps to live your dreams, and if blocks and obstacles present themselves, use them simply as an opportunity to strengthen your commitment to your dream. And make sure that you do not give current conditions of what you don't want the upper hand. If you want a loving relationship, and you are single and haven't had a date in years, keep your attention on your dream, as if it is alive in the moment. If you feel trapped in your current job, dependent on your weekly paycheck and benefits, and your dream is to start your own business, don't get lost in the drama and hopelessness you feel in your current conditions. Instead, put your energy into dreaming your new business: see it, taste it, touch it, feel it, talk about it as if it exists right now and then live into your dream in the actions you take.

HOW TO DO IT

Resource

~ *Unstoppable: 45 Stories of Perseverance and Triumph from People Just Like You* by Cynthia Kersey, Naperville, IL: Sourcebooks, Inc., 1998.

DAY 1: Articulate your dream. Imagine that it is one year from today and you are living your dream. Close your eyes and dream your life.

- Where are you living?
- Who are you living with?
- What kind of work are you doing?
- How do you feel?
- How is your health?
- How are your finances?
- How do you spend your day?
- How do you look?

Be as specific as you can, allowing your dream to enter your consciousness, and if you are uncertain of the people or places in your dream, simply allow yourself to have a sense of them.

When you have a clear sense of your dream filling your being, open your eyes and write it in your journal. On the top of the page write the date, one year from today, and begin your first sentence with: I am . . .

DAY 2: Dream twice a day. Read your dream. Make adjustments based on new ideas and information. Remember this is a fluid and evolving process. The title of this book changed four times in the midst of my writing it! Close your eyes and step into your dream. Experience it, enjoy it, fill in the details, feel a sense of excitement and satisfaction fill your being as a smile lights up your face. When you have fully dreamed your dream—this may be as quick as thirty seconds or as long as twenty minutes—ask your still small voice, "What is my next step in living my dream?" Listen to the answer and then do it. Note: It is important that you open to the loving wisdom of the universe, to that still small voice for your next step, rather than what you think you *should* do. And sometimes your next step is simply to enjoy the day!

DAY 3: Make a Dream List. Write down one hundred dreams and desires you have. Write down whatever enters your consciousness. This is not a how-to list, it is a Dream List of what your dreams are. Once you have your list written, read it and put a check ✓ next to those dreams you are ready to take action on today. For the items without a ✓, write them again on a list entitled: For The Universe to Provide—God Can. As you write each dream on this list, know that it is now in the loving hands of the universe. Have faith that the universe is at work, and your only job is to be available to receive your dream. It is okay if you put all one hundred items on this list. Our job is to express our dreams. The universe then provides, and we receive as long as we are vibrationally aligned and open to receiving, we believe we deserve it, and we trust that the universe provides what we ask for or better!

DAY 4: Create a collage of your dream. As you do this, feel your dream alive in your being. Feel the excitement in your body and the knowing in your being. Make sure to include yourself in your collage.

DAY 5: Create a dream-support buddy relationship. Share your dream with one person who has total faith in your ability to live your dreams. Ask him or her to keep you focused when and if your faith in your dreams, your faith in the universe, your faith in God, waivers.

DAY 6: Be your dream. Today have everything you think, say, and do be a reflection of you living your dream. If doubt presents itself, simply have a new thought in the next moment. What would you think, say, do, if:

- You had a great golf score?
- You had beautiful nails?
- Your marriage was delightful?
- You were in a loving relationship?
- You had financial abundance?
- You experienced well-being?
- You were an artist?
- You had your own business?
- You were living your dreams?

DAY 7: Write your reflections of your experience of focusing on and living your dreams this week.

- What did you notice?
- Do you hold back from dreaming your dreams because you are afraid you won't get them; or because you are afraid you will get them?
- Do you think you have to make your dreams happen or do you have faith in the universe to answer you call?

I do not know how to distinguish between our waking life and a dream. Are we not always living the life that we imagine we are?
—Henry David Thoreau

week 47:
Focus on Success

The Successful Self feels valuable, self-accepting and self-confident.

—DOROTHY ROWE

Focusing on success has two components. The first is how you define success, and the second is where you place your attention. Most if not all of us have grown up focusing on outside measures of success, including getting "A's" on our report card, winning a game, and living a socially acceptable life made up of marriage, children, good job, and nice home. Many people have had those successes and have not experienced peace and happiness. Peace and happiness require a definition of success that is aligned with who we are. It is an inside job that begins with listening to our heart's desire, knowing our dreams, and living our integrity. It is through this experience of being whole and aligned in our inner and outer life that we experience success.

Our ideas and beliefs about ourselves are the foundation of whether or not we experience success. If you are judgmental, self-abusive, filled with regret and shame, no matter what you achieve in the outside world, you will not feel successful. If you are self-accepting and loving, you will experience success each step of the way, honoring the journey and appreciating the destination.

In 1999 I had a powerful success experience. I had been diagnosed with uterine fibroids many years before. After a variety of treatments and remedies my acupuncturist encouraged me to schedule surgery. I decided I would approach this with all the tools I'd suggested to others. I chose a great surgeon and had a session with a psychologist who uses hypnosis in preparing patients for an easy surgery and quick recovery. I listened to audio tapes describing the skills and expertise of my surgical team and my easy and comfortable recuperation. I asked the anesthesiologist to whisper in my ear at the end of the procedure that the surgery was a success and I would heal easily and completely. I asked family and friends to pray for my highest good. The day of the surgery I felt calm and confident and focused my attention on seeing myself in my home feeling comfortable. And that is exactly what happened. I went home just two days after surgery, my recuperation was easy, and my surgeon commented on how quickly I recovered. This doesn't mean that when faced with surgery this is a prescription you should follow. Rather, it is a reminder that in being true to ourselves and marching to our own drummer, we create the opportunity for success. I concentrated on healing and used the complementary medicine that I had faith in—I focused on success. So this week explore how you define success, experiment with broadening your definitions and through your focus on success enjoy the gift of your life and be peace and happiness.

HOW TO DO IT

DAY 1: Explore what you believe about success:

1. Write your responses to the following statements: (allow all responses, free associate)
   - "Success is: _____."
   - "I am successful when I:_____."
2. After you complete your list, put a ✓ next to beliefs that support you in being successful and cross out each belief that hinders your being successful.
3. Use your marked statements as affirmations (thoughts that you affirm by repetition). Each morning and evening, read your affirmations aloud and feel the power of the words fill your being. If you hear and notice contradictory thoughts entering your mind, take a deep breath and say, "I hear you and I choose . . . (restate the affirmation with conviction and authority)." Remember you are the author of your beliefs.

DAY 2: Make a success list. On a piece of paper, in your appointment book, or in your Palm Pilot, make a list of your successes as they occur during the day. Read your list aloud at night, and allow yourself to experience your success. If you are judgmental or abusive as you read the list, go back to the beginning and read it until you go through the entire list and feel successful—feeling peace and happiness filling and embracing your being from the inside out.

DAY 3: Brag about your success. Tell three people about your experience focusing on success.

DAY 4: Make a success collage. Scissors, glue, magazines, old calendars, birthday and holiday cards that have been sent to you are the supplies you'll need. Make a collage of what success means to you and remember to include yourself in the collage; this is your success story. Hang your collage in a prominent spot, on your refrigerator or a wall filled with art of the children in your life. When you are asked about it, tell your success story.

DAY 5: Repeat the Day 1 exercise making adjustments, if necessary, to your affirmations. Randomly write your affirmations in your calendar, on the top of each page or in every few pages of your journal and on the memo section of your checks. Fill your house, office, and car with your affirmations. Put Post-It notes with affirmations written on them in places you don't see daily so you will be surprised when you see them (the inside door of your medicine cabinet, a jacket pocket, in your eyeglasses case, inside a CD holder—be creative). These are reminders to re-mind your mind about focusing on success.

DAY 6: Write a love letter to yourself about focusing on success. You may include what success is to you, a list of your successes, reminders to keep you focused on success. Put the letter in an envelope, seal it, stamp it, and give it to a friend or family member and ask him or her to mail this letter back to you at the most perfect time within the next one to two months. It will be a pleasant surprise when it arrives at the most perfect time.

DAY 7: Write your thoughts on focusing on success.

- What have you learned by focusing on success?
- What obstacles to focusing on success did you notice?
- What are your patterns of thoughts and beliefs that block your awareness of success? Knowing these patterns of thought is very powerful. When they pop up, simply say, "Oops," and choose a different train of thought to board.
- How does focusing on success contribute to your peace and happiness?
- What is your most important lesson this week?

week 48:
Sing

It is the best of all trades, to make songs, and the second best to sing them.

—Hilaire Belloc

Singing is an enjoyable way to change your mood and experience a fuller sense of peace and happiness. Singing can lift our spirits, and often the songs that pop into our minds automatically have an important message for us in the moment. Chanting, which is part of a regular Hindu spiritual practice, is used as a meditation to calm your mind and transform your experience. On occasions when I have chanted in a group for an hour, I have noticed that at some point I stop singing the chant and the chant starts singing me. My experience of myself changes, I am sound, and breath, and the experience of the words themselves. It is both a very relaxing and an energizing experience.

The power of singing has less to do with how good your voice is and more to do with your openness to allow the song to lift you and carry you on its wings. This week, experiment with singing, and create a personal song library you can use as a source of comfort, joy, peace, and happiness.

HOW TO DO IT

DAY 1: Sing. Sing in the shower, sing while you're cooking, sing while you're driving to and from your errands and work. Make up songs to sing to your pets. Sing.

DAY 2: Chant for thirty to sixty minutes. Go to your local library or music store, get a chanting tape or CD, and chant with it. Don't worry about getting each word perfectly pronounced; allow the song to lead you. If you notice your mind commenting and judging, simply focus your attention back on the sounds moving through you. One month when I was practicing chanting, I was unable to stay focused on any particular chant. I noticed that a round from my childhood, "Row, Row, Row Your Boat," kept going through my mind, so I used that when I chanted. Over and over and over again I repeated the words and they carried me gently down the stream. I realized that within this children's song, words that I had sung hundreds of times on automatic without really listening contain wisdom for living life and being peace and happiness.

DAY 3: Listen to and sing along with a kind of song that is new to you. If opera is something that is new to you, listen to great opera and allow the sounds to touch you. Don't be concerned with whether or not you understand the words. Allow the sound to speak to your heart.

DAY 4: Go to a karaoke club and sing. Again this isn't about having the best voice. This is about playing through song.

DAY 5: Put together a song library. Choose songs to calm you when you need calming, songs to inspire you, sing-alongs to sing when you're in the car with your family, songs to cook by, songs to clean by, sing-along songs when friends stop by. Remember those camp songs you sang so many years ago imprinted on your memory, sung around the campfire, sung when you were doing chores all of which created a sense of camaraderie and connection? My guess is that if you simply take a deep breath, a camp song will pop into your mind right now—sing it!

DAY 6: If singing with a group or choir is something you have always wanted to do, then join a choir, try out for your community theater musical, or take some voice lessons. Stop waiting to sing until tomorrow and do it today. My mother loved to sing. When we went to the movies, theater, or were watching a musical on TV, she would sing and hum along. When we were in public, I was embarrassed by her singing. I would lean over toward her and with annoyance in my tone, say, "Shush, Mom." She would be quiet for a moment, and then, once again, she would be captured by the song. When she was in her seventies, she joined a choir and each week sang in nursing homes. Years later, when I spoke with her about this, she told me she loved singing and had wanted to be in a choir for years. I felt so proud and inspired by Mom and learned an important lesson: it is never too late to step into our dreams.

DAY 7: Write a song that describes the power of singing in your life, and what you have learned about how singing contributes to your experience of peace and happiness.

When I wished to sing of sorrow, it was transformed for me into love.

—FRANZ SCHUBERT

week 49:
Be the World's Greatest Lover

All mankind loves a lover.

—RALPH WALDO EMERSON

Being the world's greatest lover is the leading role we were meant to play in life. While the idea of the world's greatest lover may initially evoke images of don Juan or Marilyn Monroe, I mean to include people who express love in all they think, say, and do. Since the essence of who we are is love (i.e., God is love, we are made in the image of God, therefore we are love, we are each an expression of Source Energy), each one of us has the potential to be the world's greatest lover. As great lovers, we can express our love through our sexuality as well as in our own unique way in all we think, all we say, and all we do. When we allow loving energy, Source Energy, to flow through us, everything that is not love, including anger, jealousy, envy, fear, and guilt, dissolves. Love is the force, the power that transforms everything in its path.

Too often in our lives, we put our energy and our attention into doing things, fixing things, curing things. Yet, the starting point of transforming any experience is always the presence of love, allowing Source Energy to move through our being, entering our body with every inhalation and leaving our body with every exhalation, entering our mind with every thought we give our attention to and contributing to the collective consciousness of the universe through our thoughts and words. Our feelings are our guidance system to notify us when we are out of the flow of Source Energy and love. When we pay attention to this guidance and return to love by focusing on thoughts and activities that put smiles on our faces, we can become the world's greatest lovers. This week, act as if you are the world's greatest lover and offer your love in all situations and to all people who cross your path. If you forget that being the world's greatest lover is the role you were born to play, as soon as you remember, step into that role again, loving yourself through it all. Remember being peace and happiness is another way of describing being the world's greatest lover.

HOW TO DO IT

Movies to watch and notice what happens to the characters in the presence of love:

- *Don Juan DeMarco*
- *Life As a House*
- *Shrek*
- *Beauty and the Beast*

DAY 1: Sit quietly and allow the idea of being the world's greatest lover to fill your being. You may notice sexy, graceful, sensual images come to mind. As this happens, allow your body and your being to be transformed. Feel the idea of being the world's greatest lover become alive in you. When this idea is filling your being, gently open your eyes and see the world from the vantage point of being the world's greatest lover. Repeat this exercise once an hour and notice how you feel, how you move, how you express yourself from this vantage point.

DAY 2: Write an essay entitled, "I Am the World's Greatest Lover." Read this every day and live it.

DAY 3: Imagine that the greatest sin (sin meaning being off the mark in your connection with God, with Source Energy) in the world is not expressing your love; that the greatest abuse we inflict on ourselves and others is withholding our love. With this in mind have today be a day that you are "sin free" and express your love as the world's greatest lover.

DAY 4: Make a list of the people you think are the world's greatest lovers and next to each name write down the quality of love they express. Then act as if you have those qualities. Here are some of mine:

- My mother—unconditional love for me
- Solange, my granddaughter—joy of discovering new things
- Mother Teresa—compassion
- don Miguel Ruiz—loving hug
- Jesus—forgiving heart; seeing everyone and everything as an expression of God
- Dalai Lama—contagious smile
- Catherine Zeta Jones—beauty and talent
- Sean Connery—sexy, powerful presence

DAY 5: Say "I love you" in your thoughts to every person you see or speak with today. This includes people you see on TV, in the subway, at the super-market. Notice how you feel doing this. Remember this is unconditional, independent of any circumstance or action the person is involved with, including the person talking too loudly on their cellphone; the executive who steals from his company; the trusted adult who abuses a child.

DAY 6: Create a collage that represents you as the world's greatest lover. Hang it where you can see it, and let the images of this self-portrait fill your being.

DAY 7: Write your reflections on being the world's greatest lover.

- What did you learn about yourself?
- How can you continue to be the world's greatest lover?

week 50:
Create a Bag of Tricks

*When all is said and done, each one of us is truly a bag of
tricks—a magical, mysterious creation.*

—SR

A bag of tricks is a pouch filled with good luck charms that serve as reminders of the qualities you desire to easily access. In the Native American culture, medicine bags or medicine bundles hold a collection of items that represent the medicine or power the wearer wants to have or amplify.

Since being peace and happiness requires us to have access to our personal power and consciously be able to direct it, it can be useful to have a bag of tricks to fill with lucky charms and reminders of the techniques and qualities that support peace and happiness. In a sense this book is a bag of tricks; it is filled with ideas and techniques that are entryways to peace and happiness. The more you practice the techniques and use the ideas, the easier it will be for you to consciously choose peace, happiness, and love as the energy through which you experience life. It is quite possible, though, that you might not always carry this book with you! In that case you can keep a special pouch filled with your lucky charms nearby for you to see, touch, and feel that will remind you of the power, the perspective that is always available to you for the choosing.

In addition to actually having a bag of tricks such as a pouch filled with power objects, you may already have lucky charms you wear and unconsciously reach for in times of stress. Right now, are you wearing a good luck charm? Do you have one nearby? Has one been popping into your mind as you've been reading this chapter? That special penny you always keep in your wallet; the watch that belonged to your great-grandfather and was passed on to you by your father; the rabbit's foot you keep in your sock drawer that was given to you by your favorite aunt when you were a child that makes you feel loved and safe. The special outfit you always wear when you fly on an airplane. Your wedding band that reminds you, each time you see it, that love is more important than being right in your marriage. The lucky tee that's chipped now, that you always carry in your pocket to bring you good luck on the golf course.

We can endow things with qualities and energy so they evoke a vibration, a frequency, an energy within us; or we can fill our pouch with items that are believed to have a particular meaning and vibration, and through our faith in their power we can experience a particular vibration within us. For instance, the Native American Crow tribe believed that an elk tooth was medicine that would bring material abundance to its owner; and a piece of blue cloth meant good luck.*

In addition to these good luck charms, we also call upon saints, angels, and fairies at different times in our lives to guide our way. Remember the enchanting power of the Tooth Fairy? This week, create your own bag of tricks, use it, and you will notice, as times goes by, that thoughts of your lucky charms will pop into your mind at the most perfect times and serve as regular companions and reminders for you to live your life being peace and happiness.

HOW TO DO IT

RESOURCE
_____

~ *www.vilmain.com* - sources for pewter charms

DAY 1–DAY 4: Make a list of the kinds of medicine, power, and qualities you want to have easy access to. Some of the items on your list may be:

- Health
- Abundance
- Patience
- Acceptance of self and others
- Peace
- Love
- Sense of humor
- Loving relationships

When you have completed your list, choose objects that represent each of the qualities. One way to do this is to close your eyes, focus on a specific qual-

*From Sacred Path Cards Book: *The Discovery of Self Through Native Teachings*; by Jamie Sams; 1990 Harper Collins.

ity, and ask yourself the following question: "What is a symbol of this quality?" Listen to the answer. It is possible you may not immediately get a clear
answer, but that's okay. Write the quality on a small piece of paper and trust
that the perfect symbol will be revealed to you.

Once you have chosen your objects, you will need a pouch to put them in.
You can make one, buy one, or use one you already have. This may be something you choose to wear around your neck or carry in your pocket or purse.
If you are going to make your pouch, cut your material so that the bag will be
large enough to hold your power objects and small enough to easily be carried with you. Sew your pouch. Be creative, and remember you can only do
this right. I carry a small black velvet bag of tricks in my pocketbook. It is
made from a pair of pants I loved that I had worn out. It is a bit lopsided, as
my sewing is primitive, but whenever I see it, touch it, think of it, and open
it, I feel peace and happiness.

DAY 5: Make your bag of tricks. Approach this as a sacred activity. Gather all
the items you'll need. You may listen to some lovely music, light a candle or
two, and before you jump into the task, prepare yourself by following these
instructions:

1. Make yourself comfortable.
2. Close your eyes.
3. Take a deep breath inhaling and exhaling.
4. Focus on your breath as you feel your body and mind become more
   relaxed.
5. When you experience yourself fully present in your body, state your
   intention: "I choose to create a bag of tricks that will support me in
   being peace and happiness. Each symbol I place in my pouch is a
   reminder of the qualities I always have access to."
6. Open your eyes and say aloud the "Prayer for Peace and Happiness"
   (see page 3).

Now it is time to place each item in your bag. Hold each item in your hands
one at a time (even if it is a piece of paper with the quality written on it). As
you hold it, feel the quality it represents, breathe that quality into it as you
exhale, and as you inhale receive that quality from the item. Make an agreement with each power object, asking it to remind you of its quality when you
forget and agreeing you will use its reminder to connect with the quality.

After you have made the agreement, place your power symbol in your pouch until you have agreements with each item. You now have a bag of tricks, a medicine bag. Use it, listen to it, and if you ever get the impulse to add items or remove items, do it.

DAY 6: Any time during the day when you feel off-center or in need of extra support, take out your bag of tricks and ask for the help you need. If you are unclear of what you need, ask for guidance and then reach into your bag and trust whichever power object you get is in answer to your need. Allow its quality to fill you and illuminate your way.

DAY 7: Write your reflections on creating a bag of tricks.

· What was your experience of creating a bag of tricks?
· How can you use your bag of tricks?
· What did you learn?
· What other power objects and symbols do you have and use?

Sometimes you might need to take something out of your medicine bag. I used to have a red stone, but it turned black after awhile. My Great Grandmother told me to take that stone out because it has taken on the negative energy and it was time to replace it.

—Duane Watkins

My Pocket Angel

One morning when Mom was in the intensive care unit, two months before her death, I handed her a Pocket Angel—a coin-sized, pewter charm with a lovely angel on it—and asked her to bless it. I told her I would always carry it with me and this way she would always be close to me, my special angel. It's in my wallet. I see it and touch it when I get change. Thinking of it and touching it evokes the loving embrace of Mom. It truly is a lucky charm.

—SR

week 51:
Write Your Obituary

Obituary: a notice of a person's death with a short biographical account.

—Merriam-Webster Dictionary

Writing your obituary is a powerful way to focus on what is important to you in your life. It gives you an opportunity to think about and articulate how you want the life you have lived to be described. It highlights your intrinsic values and can remind you of your priorities and heart's desires. It is a life-giving exercise focusing your intention, imagination, and actions on your vision of your life. When you do this exercise this week, don't limit yourself by what you think is possible. Open your heart and allow your imagination to do what it does best: imagine and listen to the still small voice within that answers when you ask, "What do I want said about my life when I die?" And remember, the Angel of Death is always present, so it is a good idea to live today the life you desire to live.

HOW TO DO IT

DAY 1: Still your mind:

- Sit comfortably.
- Close your eyes.
- Focus on your breath.
- Follow the path of your breath as it enters your body through your nose, circulates throughout your body, and leaves your body through your mouth. Do this for five inhalations and exhalations. Ask yourself the question, "What do I want said about the life I've lived?" Listen to the answer and write it down.

DAY 2: Make a list of what is important to you: the people, the roles you play, the activities you do. From this list, identify what truly makes your heart sing. Are these the things you currently focus on? If yes, continue. If no, choose one item on your list and begin it today.

DAY 3: Jot down phrases for your headstone. For example, "She lived well," "He lived life to the fullest," "She was the world's greatest lover," and then elaborate on what that phrase actually means to you. Allow your imagination to flow in high gear as you describe the phrase.

DAY 4: Make a collage representing the kind of life you choose to live. Allow your heart and imagination to be your guide. As you create your collage, ask yourself the question that's on my paperweight from Vilmain, Inc. "What would you do if you knew you couldn't fail?" Listen to the answer, and allow your collage to represent your heart's desire.

DAY 5: Live today as if it was your last day on earth. Make each moment count. Express your love today.

DAY 6: Write your obituary, and put it somewhere so you read it daily. This is the vision of the life you choose to create. Take time each day to see if the way you are living reflects the life you desire to live. If it does, allow yourself to feel energized, knowing the life you are living is aligned with the life you desire to live. If the life you are living and life you desire to live are at odds with each other, start making changes. Begin in your imagination seeing the life you desire, and then see it in your daily life, allowing your heart's desire to unfold, having faith that it is.

DAY 7: Write your thoughts on writing your obituary.

- What did you discover?
- How can you use this information to fully honor your life each and every day?

The Power of an Obituary

Many years ago I heard a story about Alfred B. Nobel, whose directions in his will resulted in the creation of the Nobel Peace Prize. Alfred's family was in the explosives business. When one of his brothers died, Alfred's obituary was mistakenly published in the newspaper. He read his own obituary, which highlighted his business successes describing the manufacturing of dynamite. Reading this premature obituary impelled him to change the direction of his life. Now when the name Alfred Nobel is mentioned, there is an automatic association with the Nobel Peace Prize, not with explosives!

—SR

week 52:
Create a Spiritual Practice

*The time we spend in prayer and meditation, in whatever
forms are most resonant for us, is like building spiritual
muscles. Through regular practice, we develop qualities of
strength, flexibility, endurance, and balance. We develop
wisdom, faith, equanimity, kindness; we develop deep hon-
esty and self-acceptance. We cultivate our ability to let go, our
capacity to forgive, our capacity to be present to this moment.
We learn to deeply listen, and to open ourselves to grace.*

*Then, when we need those qualities and skills in our lives,
they are there for us to draw upon and use. And our very presence may become a gift of healing, inspiration, and potential
transformation to others.*

—DIANE BERKE

Creating a spiritual practice is your opportunity to use the exercises
and techniques you have been learning, experimenting with, and
playing with this year. It is now up to you to choose the ones that resonate within your being and practice them daily. For some of you this will
look like a specific structure that you follow each day: you begin each morning with an inspirational reading, meditate for twenty minutes, and at the
end of each day write a gratitude list in your journal. Others may chant on
Monday, Wednesday, and Friday; meditate on Tuesday, Thursday, and
Saturday; and practice silence on Sunday. Others may meditate for twenty
minutes every morning and evening. There is no right or wrong way to do
this. What is important is that you do it.

Spiritual practice nourishes our connection with Source Energy, the
Loving Energy of the universe; it acknowledges that we are spiritual beings
having a human experience; it nurtures the bond between our inner experience and our outer world. And as Marianne Williamson pointed out in her
book, *Illuminata*, to go within is not to turn our backs on the world; it is to prepare ourselves to serve it most effectively.

Keep in mind that the power of spiritual practice is twofold:

1. In the midst of the practice we quiet our mind, strengthening our connection with Source Energy and experiencing the fullness of the present moment, and
2. During the course of our daily lives, because we have strengthened our spiritual muscle, we have a more direct open channel to Source Energy: love, peace, and happiness in the midst of whatever circumstances present themselves to us. When love is the lens through which we view life, magic abounds.

HOW TO DO IT

Half an hour's meditation each day is essential, except when you are busy. Then a full hour is needed.
—St. Francis de Sales

Make up a spiritual exercise plan you commit to practicing each day. Follow it for forty days. After forty days, if you want to make some adjustments and changes, do that. I have found it easier to come up with a plan and practice it long enough to get used to it, rather than make so many frequent changes that I am more focused on the changes than the practice. Forty days as a length of time comes to mind because it is the amount of time between Lent and Easter, as well as the number of years the Jews wandered in the desert. So I figure forty is a good number! Enjoy the journey and know that your peace and happiness is the biggest contribution you give to heaven on earth. Indeed, one person's peace can influence the world, as described in the following story:

Nearly twenty-two hundred years ago, about two hundred fifty years after the time of the Buddha, there lived in northern India a powerful emperor named Ashoka. During the early years of his reign, Ashoka was deeply discontent and unhappy, and greedy for the expansion of his empire. To accomplish that end, he would wage bloody and terrible wars, causing great carnage, misery, and grief.

One day, after a particularly terrible battle, Ashoka was walking on the battlefield, amid the corpses of men and animals strewn everywhere, when he was suddenly horrified by what he had caused. Just at that moment, a Buddhist monk came walking across the battlefield. The monk did not say a word, but his whole being was radiant with happiness and peace. Seeing him, Ashoka was stunned. He asked himself, "Why is it that I, who have everything, feel so empty and miserable, while this monk, who has nothing but the robes he wears and the bowl he carries, looks so serene and happy, even in this terrible place?"

Ashoka then made a momentous decision there on the battlefield. He pursued the monk and asked him, "Are you happy? If so how did that come to be?" In response, the monk, who had nothing, introduced the emperor, who had everything, to the Buddha's teachings. As a result of that chance encounter, Ashoka dedicated himself to the study and practice of Buddhism. The entire nature of his reign as emperor changed. He stopped waging imperialistic wars, he no longer let people go hungry, and he transformed himself from a cruel tyrant into a just, compassionate, and deeply respected ruler.

Ashoka's own son and daughter carried Buddhism from India to Sri Lanka, where it took root and then spread to Burma and Thailand and throughout the world. Our access to these teachings today is a direct result of Ashoka's transformation. The radiance, the serenity, of that one Buddhist monk is still affecting the world today. One person's happiness can change the course of history.

—SHARON SALZBERG, FROM *LOVINGKINDNESS: THE REVOLUTIONARY ART OF HAPPINESS*

My Spiritual Practice Testimonial

On August 11, 2002, I was driving home. I had been in New Jersey the evening before to officiate at a wedding and had spent the night in New York City. It was early in the day, and I was eager to get home and write. My manuscript was due at the publisher's on September 1, 2002, and I had plans to be out of town from August 14 to 20. I still had many chapters to write and editing to do. The roads were empty, the sun was bright and hot, and my car conked out, just as I was wondering whether or not to buy it when the lease was up in October. An orange warning light was on. I was fifty miles from home. Yuck. I pulled into a shopping mall and got the manual from the glove compartment. All I found is that when this light goes on, it means trouble. I made many phone calls: to AAA, VW Roadside Assistance, the dealer, my insurance company. By the third call, when someone at the dealer told me to get the car to them and he wasn't sure when they could look at it, I felt tears welling up in my eyes. I was thinking, "I'm covered for three miles of towing, I am fifty miles from home and forty-five miles from the dealer, which is forty miles from my house. I'm single, I live alone, I don't have another car to use, I don't know what to do, this is gonna cost a lot of money." I was in hell, and then I heard, "Everything is gonna be okay," from deep within me. This voice got my attention, as it was clear, direct, and reassuring.

Suddenly it occurred to me that I was in the midst of an adventure. My eyes dried. I decided to call my trusty local mechanic. AAA sent a tow truck. I found out my insurance would pay fifty dollars of the towing. The tow driver agreed to drive me home once we dropped my car off at my local auto shop. I remembered that friends of mine left their car at the local train station when they were in the city during the week. I called them and they said it would be fine for me to use their car. Sixteen days later, my car was repaired, and I decided to sell it before the lease was up, eliminating the charges for my extra mileage. My new car was delivered directly to my home the day after that, and my publisher did not complain about my using a few extra days to fine-tune my manuscript, especially when she heard that in the midst of my car drama, I used what I wrote about and it worked!

CHOOSE Peace & Happiness

The message of this story is that I do spiritual practice. I commune with the Loving Energy of the universe each and every day. I listen to and follow that still small voice within. I have a well-toned spiritual muscle, and through this connection with Source Energy I spend minimal time in hell. Oh yes, I step in at times, and I am tempted by the seduction of the drama, and then I quickly get a reminder that there is another way, an easier way, and I say YES and guess what? Magic happens.

—SR

184

AFTerwOrD

A s I write this, we are in the midst of war with Iraq, but we are also in the last weeks of this year's Season for Non-Violence. The Season for Non-Violence, from January 30 to April 4 each year, was initiated by Arun Gandhi (Mahatma Gandhi's grandson), his wife Sunanda, and the Association for Global New Thought on January 30, 1998, to honor the 50th and 30th memorial anniversaries of Mahatma Gandhi and Dr. Martin Luther King, Jr., respectively. The vision of this worldwide grassroots campaign is to demonstrate that non-violence is a powerful way to heal, transform, and empower our lives and our communities, and that every person can contribute to peace on earth through daily choices and actions based on compassion, respect, and understanding. The inaugural event was held at the United Nations. With the support of Secretary General Kofi Annan, the U.S. Ambassador to India, the Director General of UNESCO, and all living Nobel Peace Laureates, the United Nations unanimously declared 2001–2010 the International Decade for a Culture of Peace and Non-Violence for the Children of the World.

September 11, 2001 was the United Nations' International Day of Peace and was to have marked the beginning of the International Decade for a Culture of Peace and Non-Violence for the Children of the World. How ironic that in the midst of the tragic events that day, we were stepping into a dream of non-violence as well. I have come to know that all life is connected and intertwined. In the midst of horrific events, the call of love, kindness, peace, and compassion is often heard the loudest. And here we are today fighting a war in Iraq at the same time the call for peace is alive and expanding throughout the world. And as the war's strategy of "Shock and Awe" is described in news programs, I am seeing peace present even in the midst of fighting—with a focus on causing the least harm and following the rules of war based on the writings of Chinese philosopher and general Sun Tzu who wrote about the art of war more that 2,500 years ago.

I pray for peace, I imagine peace, I choose to live the principles of nonviolence exemplified by Mahatma Gandhi and Martin Luther King, Jr. I have faith in Gandhi's words, "Be the change you wish to see in the world." I believe in the possibility of Dr. King's "I Have a Dream" speech. And in the midst of a current reality that screams of violence, I know that the more each individual in the world lives a daily life of kindness, compassion, and love, in their homes, on line at the supermarket, in the workplace, in traffic, in the midst of personal challenges, during each moment of our day that we are changing the world.

I invite you to join me with prayers for the highest good for all beings on earth, to sign Manifesto 2000: A Vow of Non-Violence (*http://www3.unesco.org/manifesto2000/*) and to live each day following the six principles of non-violence:

- Respect all life.
- Reject violence.
- Share with others.
- Listen to understand.
- Preserve the planet.
- Rediscover solidarity.

And remember that everything in creation begins as an idea in our imagination. And then, when the idea is wedded to faith, spoken of with authority, and acted on with conviction, miracles—even the miracle of peace—are possible.

permissions

A n exhaustive effort has been made to clear all reprint permissions for this book. If any required acknowledgment has been omitted, it is unintentional. If notified, the publishers will be pleased to rectify any omission in future editions.

The author gratefully acknowledges permission to use the following material:

"Let there be peace on earth and let it begin with me" from song by Jill Jackson and Sy Miller, copyright © 1955 (renewed 1983) by Jan-Lee Music. Used by permission.

"Imagine" Words and Music by John Lennon ©1971 (Renewed 1999) LENONO MUSIC All Rights Controlled and Administered by EMI BLACKWOOD MUSIC, INC. All Rights Reserved. International Copyright Secured. Used by Permission.

Inner Peace by Elsa Joy Bailey (*www.elsajoy.com*) used by permission of the author.

Adaptation of *The Wonderful Cracked Pot* by Dan Gibson © (*www.dangibson.net*) used by permission of the author.

Rumi poem from *The Illuminated Rumi* by Coleman Barks and Michael Green, copyright © 1997, Broadway Books. Used by permission of the publisher.

"What the World Needs Now is Love" by Burt Bacharach and Hal David © 1965 (Renewed) New Hidden Valley Music and Casa David Music All Rights o/b/o New Hidden Valley Music administered by WB Music Corp. All Rights Reserved. Used by Permission of WARNER BROS. PUBLICATIONS U.S. INC., Miami, FL.

"I Heard It Through the Grapevine" Words and Music by Norman J. Whitfield and Barrett Strong © 1966 (Renewed 1994) JOBETE MUSIC CO., INC. All Rights Controlled and Administered by EMI BLACKWOOD MUSIC INC. on behalf of STONE AGATE MUSIC (A

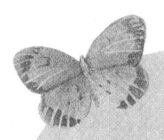

Free Gift Offer

As a thank you for
Choosing Peace & Happiness,
I'd like to offer you a free gift.

Simply go to my website at
www.susynreeve.com
and click on "Free Gift."

ABOUT THE AUTHOR

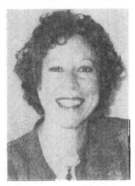

SUSYN REEVE is an ordained Interfaith Minister whose work includes organizational and personal development consulting with such organizations as NYU Medical Center, Mount Sinai Medical Center, the Plaza Hotel, Exxon, and UJA Federation. In her workshops, Susyn creates opportunities for people to identify, reconnect with, use and honor their natural resources-skills, talents, and abilities. She is co-founder of *CelebrateSomebody.com*. This is her first book. She lives in East Hampton, New York.

For more information about Susyn's:
  Workshops
  Teleclasses
  Corporate Consulting
  Mentoring & Coaching Programs
  Ceremonies
  or to book her as a Speaker
Please visit her website *SusynReeve.com* or email her at *Susyn@SusynReeve.com*.

To our Readers

Red Wheel, an imprint of Red Wheel/Weiser, publishes books on topics ranging from spunky self-help, spirituality, personal growth, and relationships to women's issues and social issues. Our mission is to publish quality books that will make a difference in people's lives—how we feel about ourselves and how we relate to one another and to the world at large. We value integrity, compassion, and receptivity, both in the books we publish and in the way we do business.

Our readers are our most important resource, and we value your input, suggestions, and ideas about what you would like to see published. Please feel free to contact us, to request our latest book catalog, or to be added to our mailing list.

Red Wheel/Weiser, LLC
P.O. Box 612
York Beach, ME 03910-0612
www.redwheelweiser.com